INTERNAL MEDICINE CLERKSHIP

150 BIGGEST MISTAKES

AND HOW TO AVOID THEM

INTERNAL MEDICINE CLERKSHIP

150 BIGGEST MISTAKES

AND HOW TO AVOID THEM

EDITED BY
Samir P. Desai, MD
Assistant Professor of Medicine, Baylor College of Medicine, Houston, Texas

AUTHORED BY
Samir P. Desai, MD, Phillip Ramos, MD, William Lee, MD,
Vaishalee Padgaonkar, Abhay Bilolikar

PUBLISHED BY

MD2B

HOUSTON, TEXAS

www.MD2B.net

The *Internal Medicine Clerkship: 150 Biggest Mistakes And How To Avoid Them* is published by MD2B, P.O. Box 300988, Houston, Texas 77230-0988

http://www.MD2B.net

NOTICE: The authors and publisher disclaim any personal liability, either directly or indirectly, for advice or information presented within. The authors and publisher have used care and diligence in the preparation of this book. Every effort has been made to ensure the accuracy and completeness of information contained in this book. The reader should understand, however, that the subject matter of the book is not rooted in scientific observation. The recommendations made within this book have come from the authors' personal experiences and interactions with other attending physicians, residents, and students over many years. Since expectations vary from medical school to medical school, clerkship to clerkship, attending physician to attending physician, and resident to resident, the recommendations are not universally applicable. No responsibility is assumed for errors, inaccuracies, omissions, or any false or misleading implication that may arise due to the text.

Printed in the United States of America

ISBN # 0-9725561-2-5

Contents

PART I: *COMMONLY MADE MISTAKES DURING—*
Prerounds

PART II: *COMMONLY MADE MISTAKES DURING—*
Work Rounds

PART III: *COMMONLY MADE MISTAKES WHILE—*
On Call

PART IV: *COMMONLY MADE MISTAKES ON—*
Write-Ups

TABLE OF CONTENTS

PART V: *COMMONLY MADE MISTAKES WHEN—*
Presenting Newly Admitted Patients

PART VI: *COMMONLY MADE MISTAKES ON—*
The Daily Progress Note

PART VII: COMMONLY MADE MISTAKES DURING—
Attending Rounds

TABLE OF CONTENTS

About the authors

Samir P. Desai, MD

Dr. Samir Desai serves on the faculty of the Baylor College of Medicine in the Department of Medicine. Dr. Desai has educated and mentored both medical students and residents, work for which he has received teaching awards.

Dr. Desai is the author of the popular *101 Biggest Mistakes 3rd Year Medical Students Make And How To Avoid Them*, a book that has helped students reach their full potential during the third year of medical school. In the book, *The Residency Match: 101 Biggest Mistakes And How To Avoid Them,* Dr. Desai shows applicants how to avoid commonly made mistakes during the residency application process.

Dr. Desai conceived and authored the Clinician's Guide Series, a series of books dedicated to providing clinicians with practical approaches to commonly encountered problems. Now in its third edition, the initial book in this series, the *Clinician's Guide to Laboratory Medicine,* has become a popular book for third year medical students, providing a step-by-step approach to laboratory test interpretation. Recent titles in this series are the *Clinician's Guide to Diagnosis* and *Clinician's Guide to Internal Medicine.*

Dr. Desai is also the founder of http://www.MD2B.net, a website committed to helping today's medical student become tomorrow's doctor. Founded in 2002, http://www.MD2B.net is dedicated to providing medical students with the tools needed to tackle the challenges of the clinical years of medical school.

After completing his residency training in Internal Medicine at Northwestern University in Chicago, Illinois, Dr. Desai had the opportunity of serving as chief medical resident. He received his MD degree from the Wayne State University School of Medicine in Detroit, Michigan, graduating first in his class.

Phillip Ramos, MD

Dr. Phillip Ramos obtained his medical degree from the Baylor College of Medicine in Houston, Texas, graduating in 2000. In 2003, he completed his residency in Internal Medicine at the Baylor College of Medicine. During the 2003-2004 academic year, he is serving as the chief medical resident at the St. Luke's Episcopal Hospital and the Houston VA Medical Center, two major teaching hospitals at the Baylor College of Medicine. During his chief year, Dr. Ramos has helped further the education of medical students, interns, and residents.

In June 2004, Dr. Ramos is scheduled to begin his nephrology fellowship at Vanderbilt University Medical Center in Nashville, Tennessee. His career goals include practicing nephrology and being a clinical educator at a major academic medical center.

William Lee, MD

Dr. William Lee obtained his medical degree from the University of Texas Medical Branch in Galveston, Texas. Like Dr. Ramos, he completed his residency in Internal Medicine at the Baylor College of Medicine in 2003 and has had the privilege of serving as the chief medical resident for the program during the 2003-2004 academic year. In June 2004, Dr. Lee will begin his nephrology fellowship at the University of Colorado Health Sciences Center. Aside from practicing nephrology, his career goals include advancing medicine and medical education.

Vaishalee Padgaonkar

Vaishalee Padgaonkar grew up in Livonia, Michigan. She completed her bachelor's degree in Cell and Molecular Biology at the University of Michigan in Ann Arbor. She was a 4th year medical student at the University of Michigan Medical School when this book was published and has plans to go on to a residency in internal medicine.

Abhay Bilolikar

As this book was being prepared for printing, Abhay Bilolikar was a 3rd year medical student at the Wayne State University School of Medicine in Detroit, Michigan. He is originally from Troy, MI and attended college at Wayne State University, where he received his Bachelor of Science degree in biology, graduating summa cum laude in 2000. Abhay has a research background of molecular biology at Wayne State University, and enjoys the challenges of tutoring and teaching. Although he is not yet sure of the specialty he plans to pursue as a career, Internal Medicine is high on the list.

Books by Samir Desai, MD

Internal Medicine Clerkship: 150 Biggest Mistakes And How To Avoid Them

The Residency Match: 101 Biggest Mistakes And How To Avoid Them

101 Biggest Mistakes 3rd Year Medical Students Make And How To Avoid Them

Clinician's Guide to Laboratory Medicine: A Practical Approach

Clinician's Guide to Laboratory Medicine: Pocket

Clinician's Guide to Diagnosis: A Practical Approach

Clinician's Guide to Internal Medicine: A Practical Approach

To view sample chapters from these books, please visit www.MD2B.net

How to Contact the Authors

MD2B provides consulting services for third and fourth year medical students. Members of the MD2B team have given talks about the pitfalls of the third year of medical school, steps to success during clinical clerkships, applying for residency, secrets to a successful Match, laboratory test interpretation made easy for the USMLE, and other topics of interest to medical students. Requests for information about consulting services, as well as inquiries about availability for speeches and seminars, should be directed to the following address:

MD2B
P.O. Box 300988
Houston, Texas 77230-0988
(713) 927-6830

Readers of this book are also encouraged to contact MD2B with comments and ideas for future editions of this book (email address info@md2b.net).

ABOUT www.md2b.net

Our website, www.md2b.net, is committed to helping today's medical student become tomorrow's doctor. Founded in 2002, www.md2b.net is dedicated to providing third and fourth year medical students with the tools needed to tackle the challenges of the clinical years of medical school.

The website provides the following information:

> Internal Medicine Clerkship survival guide
> Surgery Clerkship survival guide
> Success tips (tips of the week)
> Introduction to the residency match
> Residency match tips
> —AND MUCH MORE!

Acknowledgments

We are fortunate to have the opportunity to work with an outstanding faculty at the Baylor College of Medicine. Faculty members of the Department of Medicine that deserve special thanks for their contributions to this book include Drs. Rita Marr and Daniel M. Musher.

Preface

Every year in the United States, approximately 20,000 students rotate through the Internal Medicine Clerkship. Many of these students find the clerkship to be an overwhelming experience. Few rotations require students to learn so much in so little time. Adding to the stress is the uncertainty that accompanies the start of the clerkship. Students are often unsure of how to admit, work-up, present, and perform write-ups on patients that are assigned to them. In addition, students recognize that clinical clerkship evaluations are important in the residency application process. These concerns, which weigh heavily on the minds of students everywhere, create an environment in which mistakes can easily be made. These are the errors that prevent students from securing the best possible evaluation. For some students, the consequences of repeating these mistakes can be long lasting. In fact, they can haunt students well after medical school graduation, preventing them from reaching their full potential as physicians.

Until recently, books about clinical clerkships, including the Internal Medicine rotation, have focused entirely on educating students on what they should do. What is often left out is any discussion about the things that students should not do. With that being said, it should come as no surprise to anyone that students make the same mistakes year after year. Since students can gain valuable insight by learning about their predecessors' mistakes, we offer you this new book titled the *Internal Medicine Clerkship: 150 Biggest Mistakes And How To Avoid Them.*

This book not only introduces you to these mistakes but also shows you how to avoid them. Avoiding these pitfalls is crucial for rotation success. Once you are familiar with these errors, you can do everything in your power to avoid them, thereby placing yourself in a position to excel during the clerkship. Even if you happen to make these mistakes, this book will show you how to recover from them quickly and help you prevent them from happening again.

Readers who are familiar with the book, *101 Biggest Mistakes 3rd Year Medical Students Make And How To Avoid Them*, may wonder what the difference is between these two books. This new book essentially picks up where the other left off. Whereas the *101 Biggest Mistakes 3rd Year Medical Students Make And How To Avoid Them* offers recommendations, tips, and suggestions that are generally applicable to all rotations, the *Internal Medicine Clerkship: 150 Biggest Mistakes And How To Avoid Them* offers advice specific to the Internal Medicine Clerkship.

The detailed information that is provided in this book will help students effectively preround, shine during work rounds, deliver polished oral case presentations, develop thorough write-ups, create well-written daily progress notes, and impress the attending physician during rounds. These are the keys to securing the best possible evaluation, strong letters of recommendation, favorable Dean's letter comments, and building the foundation for a successful career as a physician. We wish you the best during the Internal Medicine clerkship and hope that this book becomes your companion, providing you with the tools needed to tackle the challenges of this rotation.

Samir Desai, MD

Phillip Ramos, MD

William Lee, MD

Vaishalee Padgaonkar

Abhay Bilolikar

How to Use This Book

What are the differences between this book and the *101 Biggest Mistakes 3rd Year Medical Students Make And How To Avoid Them*?

The *101 Biggest Mistakes 3rd Year Medical Students Make And How To Avoid Them* introduces readers to mistakes that students can make in any of the rotations taken during the third year of medical school. The book offers tips, suggestions, and recommendations to help you avoid these mistakes. These are the errors that prevent students from reaching their full potential during this important year.

In contrast, the *Internal Medicine Clerkship: 150 Biggest Mistakes And How To Avoid Them* offers rotation-specific advice for the Internal Medicine clerkship. It provides the detailed information students need to effectively preround, impress during work rounds, deliver polished oral case presentations, develop complete write-ups, create well-written progress notes, and shine during attending rounds. The information found in this book complements that which is contained in the *101 Biggest Mistakes 3rd Year Medical Students Make And How To Avoid Them.*

How do I read this book?

Although you are welcome to read this book from cover to cover, many students will find it more useful to refer to a particular chapter when the need arises. For example, before you give your oral case presentation on a newly admitted patient, you can turn to part V of this book (commonly made mistakes when presenting newly admitted patients) to educate yourself on the mistakes that your predecessors have made. The knowledge gained will help you avoid making the same mistakes.

How will I benefit from reading this book?

The mistakes contained in this book are the same mistakes we made during our Internal Medicine clerkship. Now as attending physicians and residents, we continue to see these mistakes being made by our students. We believe that students can gain valuable information from knowing about their predecessor's errors. Avoiding these pitfalls is one of the keys to building the foundation for a successful physician career—that's what the third year is all about. This book emphasizes the "nuts and bolts" of the Internal Medicine clerkship in order to help you obtain outstanding clinical evaluations and the best grade possible during your rotation.

Why are some mistakes repeated in the book?

Some mistakes are repeated because they can be made in different aspects of the rotation. For example, the chapters on the patient write-up and oral case presentation have some mistakes that they share in common. It is very common for students to avoid a mistake on the patient write-up only to make the same mistake during the oral case presentation (and vice versa). To avoid this from happening, we have repeated some of the mistakes. In addition, even when the name of the mistake is the same, keep in mind that the information in the body of the mistake may differ. Since some of these mistakes are major, repetition also serves to emphasize key points.

How do I use the appendices?

The appendices are useful supplemental sources of information that you can use during your Internal Medicine clerkship. The appendices provide you with information regarding patient data organization, (e.g. a template), EKG/CXR interpretation, and other general pearls of wisdom to help you succeed in this clerkship.

Prerounds

During the Internal Medicine Clerkship, your day will typically begin with prerounds. During prerounds you will see your patients alone. The goal is to identify any new events that have occurred in your patient's course after you left the hospital on the previous day. The information that you gather will be presented to the resident and intern during work rounds (morning rounds), which immediately follow prerounds. In this chapter we will discuss commonly made mistakes during prerounds.

Mistake # **1**

Setting aside too little time for prerounds

The amount of time you will need to preround will vary based on a number of factors. Early in the rotation, you may need more time because of unfamiliarity with the new rotation and its responsibilities. As you become comfortable in your setting, you will become more efficient and require less time for prerounding. Other considerations are the number of patients you are following and the complexity of the cases. Be sure to give yourself enough time because if you are rushed it will be difficult to do your best work.

Success tip # 1

Arrive early. Give yourself enough time to see your patients and gather the necessary information without being rushed. An extra cushion of time is especially helpful when the patient had an eventful night, in which case there may be considerable information to gather and sort through. Allow ample time for the unexpected.

Mistake # <u>2</u>

Not knowing what to do during prerounds

The goal of prerounds is to identify any new events that have occurred in your patient's course after you left the hospital on the previous day. During prerounds, you must complete the tasks listed in the following box.

What to do during prerounds

- Review the chart for any new progress notes (including nursing and consultant's notes) that may have been placed after you left the hospital

- Review the patient's orders, looking for any new orders that may have been written after you left the hospital

- Talk with the intern (i.e., cross covering intern) who was taking care of your patient while your team was out of the hospital to see if any new events have occurred in your patient's hospital course. If this is not possible, make sure you touch base with your intern who will get sign-out from the cross covering intern.

- Talk with the nurse who was involved in your patient's care to see if they have any concerns or issues about the patient.

- Talk with the patient. You should try to ascertain the following:

   - Has the patient's overall condition improved, stayed the same, or worsened?

   - Does the patient still have the same symptoms? If so, have the symptoms improved, stayed the same, or worsened?

   - Does the patient have any new symptoms?

   - Does the patient have any new concerns? Questions?

- Examine the patient. You should do the following:

continued next page

2

What to do during prerounds, continued

- Write down the most recent vital signs (BP, HR, RR, temperature), maximum temperature (Tmax), O_2 sat (if pertinent), weight (if pertinent), blood glucose checks (if pertinent), and Ins/Outs (if pertinent). Also note any trends in the temperature, BP, or HR. If vital signs have not been done recently, do them yourself.
- Check the IV. Make note of the type of intravenous fluids hanging and the rate of administration.
- Perform a brief physical exam: focus on the area of interest (for example, if the patient has a foot ulcer, take a look at the foot!) At a minimum, you should also perform a heart, lung, abdomen, and lower extremity exam, irrespective of the reason for the hospitalization.
- Check to see if lab/diagnostic test results have returned (labs, EKG, radiographs, etc.)
- Gather your thoughts and formulate your assessment and plan for each problem.
- Get ready to present this information to the resident and intern during work rounds.

Mistake # <u>3</u>

Information gathered during prerounds is not written down

The information that you gather during prerounds will be presented to your resident and intern during work or morning rounds, which immediately follow prerounds. You will also need this information when you write the patient's progress note. For these reasons, it is important to write down the information (see box in Mistake # 2). Be sure to organize the information so that it is readily available to you

---

Success tip # 2

Write down any information you gather during prerounds because you will need to convey this information to your resident and intern during work rounds (rounds with resident and intern). You will also need to refer to it when you write the patient's progress note.

Mistake # 4

Chart is not reviewed for new progress notes

Progress notes may be placed in the chart after you leave the hospital. Because consultants and attending physicians often round late, their notes may not make it into the chart until late in the day. When you are prerounding, one of your first activities should be to read through the progress notes to get up to speed on your patient's condition.

Success tip # 3

A review of the chart for any new progress notes is a must. It is one of the keys to getting up to speed on your patient's hospital course. Read all new progress notes, including those left by the nurses.

Success tip # 4

Before leaving the hospital for the day, consider catching up on any new progress notes that may have been added to the chart. This will shorten the amount of time you need for the next day's prerounds.

Mistake # 5

Chart is not reviewed for new orders

New orders may be written after you leave the hospital. These orders may have been written by the patient's attending physician, consultant, or cross-covering intern. Quite often, they are not documented in the progress notes. Therefore, important information may be missed unless you look at the orders. Review of the orders will also allow you to determine if recommendations made by consultants were implemented. It is not sufficient to simply make note of any new orders. You should try to determine why the order was written. If it is unclear, be sure to ask the intern.

Mistake # 6

Not talking with the cross-covering intern

After you and your team have completed your work and left the hospital, the care of your patients will be transferred to the cross-covering intern. It is the cross-covering intern who will be called to evaluate and treat the patient should his or her condition change in any way. Sometimes, the patient's condition may change dramatically in which case the cross-covering intern may have to do quite a bit for your patient. In other cases, it may be as simple as the nurse calling the cross-covering intern to ask him or her to prescribe a sedative for your patient if he or she is having difficulty sleeping.

Be sure to talk with the cross-covering intern to learn if he or she had to do anything for your patient while you and your team were away. At most places, however, students do not have access to the cross-covering intern. What typically happens is that the cross-covering intern will report directly to the intern on your team who is also taking care of your patient. Thus, your intern may be well informed but you may find yourself out of the loop. If the cross-covering intern is not accessible to you, touch base with your own intern to find out what, if anything, the cross-covering intern had to do for your patient

---

Success tip # 5

Your intern may know things about your patient that you do not. Remember that he or she will receive report (sign-out) from the cross-covering intern who was taking care of your patient while you and your team were out of the hospital. Always ask your intern if he or she knows anything about your patient that you are not privy to.

Mistake # 7

Not having the vital signs information

Nurses measure blood pressure, heart rate, respiratory rate, and temperature periodically in hospitalized patients. These vital signs are usually recorded on a bedside chart or flowsheet. Information about total intake and output (I & Os), finger stick blood glucose (blood glucose checks over the past 24 hours), urine output, oxygen saturation (pulse ox), and drainage from any surgical drains or chest tubes may also be reported.

For the purposes of work rounds, you must have the patient's most recent vital signs. If vital signs have not been performed in a while, do them yourself. You should also have the Tmax (maximum temperature over the past 24 hours) and any important vital sign trends. Depending upon the reason for hospital admission, you may have to weigh the patient if nursing has not already done so.

Mistake # 8

Focused physical exam is not performed

While students are expected to perform complete physical exams at the time of admission, there is no need to do so during prerounds. Here, the goal is to perform focused physical exams. Always focus on the areas of interest. For example, if the patient has a foot ulcer, you clearly want to look at the foot. In addition, you must perform a heart, lung, abdomen, and lower extremity exam on every patient, irrespective of the complaint that prompted their hospitalization.

Success tip # 6

You must perform a heart, lung, abdomen, and lower extremity exam on every patient, irrespective of the reason for the patient's hospitalization.

Mistake # 9

Forgetting to see if lab or diagnostic test results have returned

Hospitalized patients often have daily blood draws, which are usually done early in the morning. Laboratory test results may become available during prerounds. Although these results will often be placed in the patient's chart, there is usually a window of time during which test results are available in the computer but have not found their way into the chart. For this reason, always check the computer for up-to-date lab test results.

You should know what was ordered, what has returned, and what is pending. Also do not forget that some tests may have been ordered days ago (e.g. blood cultures) but take time to return. Do not forget about these pending lab test results. Having a system in place that reminds you of pending lab test results is recommended.

Success tip # 7

Always check the computer for the most up-to-date lab test results. Do not rely on the chart because it often takes some time for the most recent results to make their way to the patient's chart.

Mistake # **10**

Not giving yourself enough time to gather your thoughts before work rounds

Up until now, all you have done is gather information. The whole point of this is to get ready for work rounds, which will immediately follow prerounds. During work rounds your team will expect you to present this information to them. In addition, they expect to hear your thoughts about the patient's assessment and plan. To develop the assessment and plan, you need to carefully consider the information you have gathered. This will allow you to make recommendations regarding diagnostic testing and management. Since this requires some thought, be sure to give yourself enough time to formulate the assessment and plan.

Success tip # 8

You must think about the data that you have gathered. Actively processing the data will help you formulate an assessment and plan.

Work Rounds

During work rounds, also known as morning or resident rounds, the team (usually without the attending physician) travels from room to room, seeing each of the patients on the service. At times, depending on the institution, other healthcare professionals (dieticians, pharmacist, nurse, social worker, etc.) may join rounds. The most junior member of the team (junior medical student, senior medical student, intern), who is following the patient, is required to update the team on the patient's progress. This update will include any significant events that have occurred overnight and the results of any lab/diagnostic testing. The information you present will help the team formulate a diagnostic and therapeutic plan. Commonly made mistakes during work rounds are discussed in this chapter.

Mistake # **11**

Not knowing your resident's expectations for you during work rounds

Early in the rotation, you must meet with your resident to learn about what he or she expects from you during the rotation. During this meeting, the resident may inform you about your responsibilities during work rounds. If he or she does not volunteer this information, be sure to ask. The way work rounds are conducted varies from one resident to another. That is why it is important to know about your resident's preferences. Questions to ask your resident about work rounds are included in the following box.

Questions to ask about work rounds

Where will work rounds begin?

What information should I gather for work rounds?

continued next page

Questions to ask about work rounds, continued

What time does work rounds start?
How much time do I have for my work rounds presentation?
How would you like me to present newly admitted patients during work rounds?
How would you like me to present old or established patients during work rounds?
In what order should I present the information?
How detailed should my work rounds presentation be?

Usually you will be asked to present your patients to the team during work rounds. The information that you convey updates the team on your patient's hospital course. It allows the team to develop a plan for the day (e.g., further diagnostic testing, changes in management, etc.).

Mistake # **12**

Showing up late for work rounds

Although the time at which work rounds start varies from one institution to another, at most places, work rounds immediately follow prerounds. Common times at which work rounds start include 7 AM, 7:30 AM, and 8 AM. The time may also vary, depending upon the patient census.

In most Internal Medicine clerkships, you will be asked to preround before work rounds. If you do not give yourself enough time to preround, you may be late for work rounds, in which case you will hold up the team. Since there is much to do during work rounds, your resident and intern will not be pleased if you are late.

Success tip # 9

Always be on time for work rounds. There is much to do and if you are late, the team will be behind schedule.

Mistake # 13

Not being brief

Oral patient presentations during work rounds are expected to be brief. There simply isn't enough time for long-winded presentations. After all, the entire service of patients must be seen during the time allotted for work rounds. At most institutions, the team is given 1 to 1.5 hours to complete work rounds. When the size of the service is large, it can be a challenge to see and discuss each patient within this time period. For example, if there are 20 patients on the service, only three minutes are available per patient if work rounds are to be finished in 60 minutes. For this reason, brief oral patient presentations are a must.

Success tip # 10

Brief oral patient presentations are preferred during work rounds. Ask your resident how much time you have to present the information. Do not exceed the time allotted to you.

Mistake # 14

Being unfamiliar with the order of the work rounds presentation

As stated in mistake # 11, it is important to ask your resident about any preferences he or she may have in terms of the order in which you present patient information during work rounds. Most residents expect that you will use the SOAP format (subjective, objective, assessment, plan) for the work rounds presentation. This is essentially the same order that you will use when writing the patient's progress note. A step-by-step guide to the work rounds presentation is described in the following box.

11

Step by step approach to the work rounds presentation

Step 1: Start your work rounds presentation with a short summary of the patient to remind the team of his or her problems. Present the patient to the team by giving the patient's name, age, gender, and chief complaint or working diagnosis/reason for being in the hospital

> *Example: Mr. Smith is a 64-year old white male who was admitted two days ago with shortness of breath and diagnosed with COPD exacerbation.*

Step 2: Present the subjective data, which should include the patient's current status and any events/complaints that have occurred or developed since yesterday's rounds.

> *Example: He states that his night was uneventful. He continues, however, to have shortness of breath without significant improvement from the day of admission. He denies fever, cough, or chest pain.*

Step 3: Present the objective data, beginning with the most recent vital signs (temperature, blood pressure, heart rate, respiratory rate, and pulse oximetry [mention the amount of oxygen patient is receiving]). Also mention the maximum temperature in the last 24 hours. Express the vitals in regards to ranges as well. Also mention the total fluid input and output, blood glucose checks over the last 24 hours, and daily weights if pertinent to the patient.

> *Example: Current respiratory rate, pulse, temperature, and blood pressure are 18, 84, 99, and 130/80, respectively. Maximum temperature (Tmax) of 99. The blood pressure has ranged from 118/75 to 185/95.*

continued next page

Step by step...work rounds presentation, continued

Step 4: Present the physical exam findings from your most recent exam. In addition to always presenting the heart, lung, abdominal, and lower extremity exam (be brief!), also include findings pertinent to the patient's problem (for example, your resident will want to know about the patient's foot ulcer if that's why the patient was admitted).

> *Example: Physical exam is remarkable for prolonged expiratory phase and scattered expiratory wheezes throughout both lung fields. Heart exam reveals a regular rate and rhythm. Abdominal and lower extremity exams are unremarkable. The rest of his physical exam is unchanged from the admission exam.*

Step 5: Present the laboratory test results. Include only new lab test results (if they are back yet). Present pertinent or changed lab values, not unchanged or normal values. Old results may be presented if needed as a reference point.

> *Example: All laboratory test results are normal except for the serum BUN and creatinine, which are 30 and 1.5, respectively. Admission values were 15 and 1.0, respectively.*

Step 6: Present the results of any other diagnostic studies or imaging tests. Include only the results of new studies or tests.

> *Example: Chest x-ray performed yesterday revealed no evidence of pneumonia or pneumothorax*

continued next page

13

Step by step...work rounds presentation, continued

Step 7: Discuss each of the patient's problems in descending order of importance. Provide an assessment for each problem followed by the management plan.

> *Example: Problem # 1 is COPD exacerbation. He has been receiving albuterol and atrovent nebs every 8 hours. Despite this therapy, his condition has not improved. The plan is to increase the frequency of the neb treatments to q4 hours and add intravenous solumedrol at a dose of 60 mg q6 hours. I'll continue to check in on him every few hours.*
>
> *Problem # 2 is HTN. He has been normotensive over the past 24 hours. The plan will be to continue his antihypertensive regimen of hydrochlorothiazide and felodipine.*

Mistake # 15

Not bringing the EKG or x-ray with you

If an EKG or x-ray (or other study) is done on your patient after you leave the hospital, bring it with you to work rounds. During rounds, your intern and resident can review the study. This will save them from making a trip to the radiology or cardiology department later. In addition, decisions regarding patient management will not be delayed.

Success tip # 11

If possible, bring any new studies (e.g., EKG, x-ray) with you to work rounds. If you bring the study to them, you will save the resident and intern some time, thereby increasing the efficiency of the entire team. Do not forget to bring the old studies with you for comparison.

Mistake # **16**

A to-do list is not made

During work rounds, your resident may ask you to take care of a number of things. It is in your best interests to write everything down. Making a to-do list will help you organize your day and make you more efficient. As you complete each task, you can cross it off your list. Do not try to memorize the tasks that need to be completed—that is a recipe for disaster. You may not be lauded for getting everything done, but your resident or intern will be disappointed and upset if you forget to do something.

Success tip # 12

On a daily basis, your resident may assign you patient-care tasks. Make sure you write these down. After work rounds, make it a habit to review the to-do list with your intern to make sure you have everything that needs to be done. Do not rely on your memory because if you forget to do something, your resident will have to answer to the attending physician.

Mistake # **17**

Tasks that need to be completed are not prioritized

During work rounds, a plan of action will be developed for each of your patients. This plan may involve a variety of tasks, including laboratory testing, performing studies, and requesting consultations. Some of these tasks are clearly more important than others. The importance of each of these tasks is something that you will have to ascertain from talking with your resident and intern. Tasks that are of higher priority should be tackled first. In addition, some tasks will not be done that day unless you tackle them early. For example, if you fail to call consults and order diagnostic testing early in the day, they are unlikely to be done until the following day.

Mistake # **18**

Orders are not written during work rounds

In general, you should write the daily orders on every patient you are following. Since the plan for the day will be formulated during work rounds, this is an ideal time to write the patient's orders in the chart. If this is not possible, write them immediately after work rounds. After you have written the orders, you can have the resident or intern cosign them. Once your orders have been cosigned, they can be implemented.

Success tip # 13

Make it a habit to write the patient's orders during work rounds. That way, there will be no delay in the implementation of the day's plan. If you wait until later, you may waste valuable time searching for your intern or resident. Without a physician's signature, orders cannot be implemented.

Mistake # **19**

The plan is not understood

The assessment and plan are the two most difficult parts of the work rounds presentation. Do your best to formulate an assessment and plan on your own. Do not be surprised, however, if your resident disagrees with or modifies your assessment and plan. You are not expected to be proficient with the development of the assessment and plan. It is more important to show the resident that you have thought about the things that are going on with your patient and that you have tried to formulate a plan based on consideration of these things. If you are having problems formulating a plan, review the plan with your intern prior to work rounds. Formulating a plan during work rounds and refining it with your team members will help you present a better plan with your attending physician later in the day.

Success tip # 14

Your intern and resident like to hear your own plans because it reflects your thinking process. Do not defer to the intern to say the plan. This is your patient, so try your best to offer a plan. It clearly shows initiative on your part and with practice and time, the development of the assessment and plan will become easier.

It is common for students to not understand the plan. For example, during work rounds, your resident may ask you to order lab test X and start medication Y. It may not be apparent to you why lab test X was ordered or why medication Y was started. If it is not clear, it is important to ask your resident or intern why you are doing what you are doing. Since this is your patient, you obviously want to have a firm understanding of the diagnostic and therapeutic plan. In addition, attending physicians commonly ask students about the plan in an effort to determine the student's depth of understanding of the patient's medical problems.

Mistake # **20**

Not paying attention during work rounds

Work rounds is an ideal time for teaching and many residents take this opportunity to show students interesting physical findings, discuss lab test results, review imaging test results, and make management decisions. Because residents can often predict what an attending physician may ask students during attending rounds, it is important to pay close attention to the things that are said during work rounds (on all of the patients not just the ones that you are following!). The pearls of information, tips, and questions that come up during work rounds may very well come up again during attending rounds. If they do, you will be able to provide the correct answers, which will leave your attending physician with a very favorable impression.

Success tip # 15

Residents often teach during work rounds. Listen to your resident when he or she tries to teach you something. Quite often, they will pass along important pearls of information, which may very well be the answers to your attending physician's questions.

Success tip # 16

Be enthusiastic during work rounds. Show your resident and intern your interest by asking questions and paying attention. Listen to all patient presentations and discussions even though you may not be directly following the patient(s). Residents do not appreciate indifferent, unenthusiastic students who are not interested in what they are doing.

Success tip # 17

Answering questions during work rounds is not an opportunity to compete and "show up" your medical student classmates. Residents and interns do not like it when students do this. This shows them you are NOT a team player, and that you care more about your grade than your classmates.

Mistake # **21**

Going to morning report when there is unfinished business

Morning report is a conference where residents present and discuss cases that they have encountered. The format may vary, but generally a resident is asked to present an interesting case, while another resident, who is unfamiliar with the case, dissects the case. As the name suggests, this conference takes place sometime in the morning, often right after work rounds and just before attending rounds. If you talk to residents, many of them will tell you that morning report is one of their favorite conferences of the day. Although this conference is directed at the intern and resident level, it can be a wonderful learning experience for students as well. However, it may not be in your best interests to attend when there is unfinished business.

For example, during the rotation, you will find that most of your mornings are spent rounding. After rounding on each patient, you will usually develop a checklist of things "to do." While some of these "to do" tasks can be done later in the day, others need to be done as soon as possible, or else patient care may be compromised or the patient's discharge may be delayed. Going to morning report instead of taking care of these tasks will not only affect patient care, but will also affect the evaluation of your performance by the resident.

Another type of unfinished business is not being prepared for attending rounds. If you did not have time to read about your patient's problems or you have not put all the pieces of the puzzle together regarding your patient's care, then you need to do this before attending rounds.

On Call

During your Internal Medicine clerkship, you will be accepting new admissions with your ward team. "On call" denotes the time you are admitting new patients onto the service. Call structure varies according to the medical institution, but in general, ward teams will admit anywhere from 5-10 patients when on call. Call can either be during the day or night. Being on call is an excellent time to work-up new, interesting patients, and to spend time with your team. This chapter reviews common mistakes made by medical students during call.

Mistake # <u>22</u>

Being unfamiliar with your on call responsibilities

If you have never been on call before, unfamiliarity with your on call responsibilities is certainly to be expected. Even if you have been on call on other clerkships, keep in mind that the on call experience and responsibilities will vary from one rotation to another. In addition, residents and attending physicians may have their own preferences. For these reasons, at the beginning of the rotation, check with your resident and attending physician to learn about what is expected of you when you are on call. Find out from them what you need to do when you evaluate a new patient.

Typically, a student will be assigned 1-2 new patients per call. Generally, you will be responsible for performing a history and physical exam, gathering the results of laboratory/diagnostic testing, presenting your findings to the intern/resident, and writing up the history and physical exam. By no means is this an exhaustive list but just a brief description of some of the tasks you need to tackle while on call. This chapter will discuss these tasks as well as other responsibilities in more detail.

Mistake # 23

Not being adequately prepared for your call

It is not surprising that many students find their first on call experience during the Internal Medicine clerkship to be quite stressful. Some even describe it as intimidating and frustrating. You can reduce a lot of this stress by being familiar with your on call responsibilities (see Mistake # 22). In addition, having everything you need to successfully complete a call can make a major difference. Start by placing items that you need in an on call bag that you will bring to the hospital. In this bag, you can have a change of clothes and personal hygiene items. Most students also recommend having snacks (food and beverages) on hand because call may be so busy that you are not able to get food from the hospital cafeteria before it closes. Of course, it is also important to bring any books or resources you need to work-up newly admitted patients.

Mistake # 24

Essential patient information is not obtained before the patient is seen

Before seeing the patient, be sure to have the patient's name, medical record number, and location in the hospital (e.g., emergency room or nursing unit). Obtain this information from your resident when he or she gives you an admission. Without this information, it will be difficult to start your admission work-up. For example, you need the patient's name and medical record number to access the patient's medical files and other important information, such as lab studies and imaging test results. Knowing the reason for the patient's hospitalization (i.e., chest pain rule out myocardial infarction) is also very helpful because if you are unfamiliar with the work-up or illness, you can quickly read about it. This will help you know what to ask when obtaining the patient's history of present illness.

Success tip # 18

When the resident informs you of a new patient admission, begin by writing the patient's essential information on the material you are using to follow your patients, such as a patient card or a note-card. Remember to always have the patient's full name, medical record number, and location with you because this information is commonly needed to access vital information and to request tests.

Mistake # 25

Patient is not seen in a timely fashion

After a patient has been assigned to you, see the patient and perform the history and physical as soon as possible. The admitting process is a busy time for your patient. The goal is to evaluate the patient, determine a plan, and write admission orders so the patient can be started on his or her treatment regimen without delay. Also, try not to take too long to evaluate the patient. This will slow down the team and frustrate the resident, who is trying to begin therapy for the patient's illness as soon as possible.

Mistake # 26

Not knowing the approach to evaluating a new patient

There are many ways to evaluate a new patient. One of the more efficient ways is to review previous records to access background information before seeing the patient. This review may provide you with information on how the patient has been and what has been done during previous hospitalizations. This information is certainly of importance in gaining a complete understanding of the patient's current clinical presentation and illness. Depending on your institution and your team, however, you may be asked to evaluate a new patient from scratch, without having any of the patient's background information. The following approach outlines a technique often used to ensure that medical students learn how to perform an evaluation on a newly admitted patient. Even if old charts or records are not available, you can still use this approach. Just skip over the steps that mention the use of charts.

Evaluating the New Patient When On Call

Step 1: Have a patient information template available to collect all patient data. We have provided a sample patient data template in Appendix H. Use this or something similar to record all of your patient information. Having the data on the template will help you organize the information for write-ups and oral case presentations.

Step 2: Check to see if there are previous medical records on your patient. If there are, look them over and see if they contain any information that is relevant to the patient's current reason for hospitalization. In some hospitals, you have to call and request medical records. It may take some time before the records are pulled, so a good approach is to call for the records and then go to Step 3.

Step 3: Before seeing the patient, review the emergency room or clinic notes, which prompted the admission.

Step 4: See the patient and perform a *complete* history and physical.

Step 5: Gather lab test results, EKGs, and imaging test results. Remember to write these results in your patient template.

Step 6: Afterwards, review and organize the information. Consult books and other resources to help you formulate an assessment and plan. Ask yourself the following questions:

- What is the most likely diagnosis and why?
- What is the differential diagnosis?
- What further evaluation is needed to support my working (likely) diagnosis?
- What treatment should I recommend?

continued next page

Evaluating the New Patient When On Call, continued

The answers to these questions will help you create your own assessment and plan.

Step 7: Present the information and offer your assessment and plan to the resident. Use the information from your patient template to help you present an organized H&P. Do not forget to ask the resident for feedback, especially about your assessment and plan.

Step 8: Write the admission orders following the format given in Mistake # 32. Remember to have your intern or resident review and co-sign all orders.

Mistake # 27

Patient's medical records are not obtained or reviewed

Hospitalized patients may have had previous hospital admissions, often at the same hospital. If they have had a previous admission, ask the medical records department for the patient's records. To locate the records, you will need to provide the patient's name and medical record number. At some institutions, medical records may be available electronically, in which case you may be able to access the information from any one of the institution's computer stations. Keep in mind that older records may not be available electronically in which case you should ask the medical records department to locate them.

Obtaining the patient's medical record at the time of admission is extremely helpful for gathering information, particularly if the patient you are admitting cannot give a reliable history. The medical record will have previous admission H&Ps, discharge summaries, EKGs, and imaging studies that may be pertinent to the current admission. For example, if a patient with coronary artery disease presents with chest pain, previous discharge summaries may reveal that he had a normal cardiac catheterization study one year ago. Pertinent information of this sort can certainly impact your assessment and plan.

Success tip # 19

Patients are usually unable to remember everything about their medical history, so having information from the medical record, when available, can be extremely useful for filling in the gaps.

Mistake # **28**

ER or clinic notes are not reviewed

Prior to seeing the patient, review the ER or clinic notes from the current visit to gather information about the admission. In addition to the patient's current complaint, these notes will offer some insight into why the patient is being hospitalized. These notes may also contain lab test results, EKGs, and imaging test results. Since treatment is often started before the patient is hospitalized, these notes will inform you of these therapies (i.e., medications, intravenous fluids).

Success tip # 20

Know what has been done for the patient in the ER or clinic prior to your involvement in his or her care. Be familiar with the evaluation performed there, including the lab/diagnostic studies obtained and the medications/ therapies that were administered. In order to provide the best possible care, it is essential that you know this information. It is likely that your attending physician will ask for this information during your oral case presentation.

Mistake # **29**

A complete history and physical exam is not performed

This is the medical student's opportunity to perform a complete history and physical. Thus, you should cover all aspects of the history, including a complete review of systems. Attempt to do a thorough physical examination, including ophthalmoscopic, otoscopic, and rectal examinations (when appropriate). If you are unsure how to perform certain aspects of the physical examination, ask your intern or resident before attempting it. Your resident and attending physician will not be pleased if you skip a particular component of the physical exam because you did not feel it was necessary. As a third year medical student, you simply do not have the experience or knowledge to determine what is and is not necessary. Therefore, it is in your best interests to perform a complete physical examination. Not uncommonly, a thorough history and physical exam performed by a student will discover something that the resident and intern may have missed.

Success tip # 21

Remember to document all vital signs from admission. Document the blood pressure, heart rate, temperature, respiratory rate, and if the patient is requiring oxygen, pulse oximetry. If the vital signs have not been performed, do them yourself. You will be asked for admission vital signs when giving your oral case presentation.

Mistake # <u>30</u>

Forgetting to gather information from studies done on admission

During the evaluation of your patient, remember to obtain the results of all studies done on admission. This includes lab test results, EKGs, and imaging test results. Lab test results and EKGs may be found in the ER or clinic chart prior to admission. X-rays may be stored in the radiology file room. Collecting this data helps your team tremendously because it saves time and increases efficiency.

Success tip # 22

Interpret the studies on your own first. Then ask your intern or resident to review the studies with you. Also, review any imaging tests with the radiologist so you have a better understanding of the findings.

Mistake # **31**

Not thinking about your assessment and plan after evaluating the patient

After evaluating the patient, many medical students are tempted to present all the data to the resident without giving any thought to the problem list, assessment, and plan. Remember, your resident is evaluating your thought process and problem-solving skills. Thus, before presenting your H&P, review the patient's data and formulate a thorough problem list. Then, make an assessment and plan for each problem.

Success tip # 23

Remember that your resident must also perform a history and physical on the patient. Presenting an organized and concise admission H&P to your resident helps him formulate his own assessment and plan. Providing your own thoughts regarding the assessment and plan will impress your resident.

Success tip # 24

Whenever possible, try to read about your patient's chief complaint and illness before presenting to your resident. This will help you prepare for any questions about the patient's disease process or plan.

Success tip # 25

If time permits, present the case to the intern. The intern may provide you with tips and hints on what the resident or attending physician may ask you about your patients.

Mistake # 32

Relying on your intern to write the patient's admission orders

You should be involved as much as possible in the evaluation and management of the patient's illness. This includes writing of the admission orders. This will not only help you understand the plan better but it also helps lighten the workload on your busy intern. If you do not understand the patient's plan, have the intern or resident write the admission orders with you. After writing the admission orders, remember to have the resident or intern review and co-sign them.

The following table contains a popular mnemonic to help you remember the contents of the admission orders. (ABC-VANDALISM)

Admitting Orders Mnemonic

Admit to (location, what service)

Because (admitting diagnosis/problems)

Condition (good, fair, critical)

Vitals (parameters, frequency, pulse-oximetry)

Allergies (medication allergies)

Nursing (blood glucose checks, foley to gravity, strict I/Os, daily weights, precautions)

Diet

Activity

Labs (e.g., CBC in the AM)

IVF (if not giving fluids, write down "saline-lock IV")

Studies (e.g., EKG in the AM, CT Scan of the Chest)

Medications

Mistake # 33

Not notifying your resident when the patient is seriously ill

The clinical status of a hospitalized patient can change quickly. If a patient appears seriously ill when you first see him or if the patient takes a turn for the worse during your evaluation, CALL YOUR RESIDENT IMMEDIATELY. Do not wait until you present your H&P to the resident to inform him of the patient's serious status.

As an example, consider a patient admitted into the hospital from the ER with suspected pyelonephritis. Over the phone, the patient was described by the ER staff to your resident as being alert, hemodynamically stable, and only complaining of right flank pain. You are the first member of your team to see the patient, and you find the patient tachypneic, confused, hypotensive, and tachycardic. Clinically, this patient is now in septic shock and requires immediate volume resuscitation and transfer to the intensive care unit.

If you encounter a patient with active chest pain, shortness of breath, confusion, unresponsiveness, hypotension, or just appears sick, be safe and call your resident to assess the patient immediately. Do the same if you encounter severely abnormal lab test, EKG, or imaging test results.

Mistake # 34

Discussing with the patient or family issues you are unsure of

Sometimes patients and their families regard medical students as physicians. Thus they may ask medical students specific questions about the treatment plan or prognosis of the patient. Even if you know the answers it is in your best interest to defer answers to these questions to your intern or resident. You certainly do not want to unintentionally mislead the patient.

Mistake # 35

Not obtaining patient information from other potential sources

If you are unable to obtain a reliable history from the patient, do not stop there! Attempt to contact family members who may be able to provide the information you need. If the patient lives in a nursing home, call the nursing home and speak to the caregivers. If the patient was recently discharged from another hospital, call the medical records department at that hospital to have the discharge summary sent to you. Do not simply defer these tasks to the intern. Interns are busy and usually do not have as much time as you do to look up these phone numbers and make the necessary calls.

Success tip # 26

You can sometimes find the patient's contact information in the hospital medical record. This contact person may be a family member, caregiver, or someone else who can provide information regarding the patient. Remember to write down the family member or caregiver's home, work, and cell phone numbers. Write down their names and contact information in your patient card template.

Mistake # 36

Not offering to help the team before leaving

Medical students are often the first ones to finish since they have fewer patients and less responsibility for patients. When you complete your work, do not just leave without offering to help other team members. The on call day is busy and stressful for the entire team. Any assistance that you can provide the resident or intern will be appreciated. This is one way to show that you are a team player. If you are a team player, your resident and intern will make more of an effort to teach you. Your clerkship evaluation will also be much more positive.

Success tip # 27

Before leaving the hospital, make sure that all orders written for the patient have been implemented. For example, check to see if the patient is receiving the fluids and medications you have prescribed. Often, the intern will do this but if he or she is too busy, there may not be time to do so. If you can take care of this responsibility, not only will you improve patient care but you will also decrease your intern's workload.

Write-Ups

The write-up or written case presentation is a detailed account of the patient's clinical presentation. You were probably introduced to the process of writing a case presentation during your physical diagnosis course. During the Internal Medicine clerkship, you will be asked to do write-ups on patients you admit. One of the major purposes of the write-up is to help you develop the written communication skills needed to take care of patients. These are skills that will serve you and your patients well throughout your medical career. For many attending physicians, the oral case presentation and patient write-up are two major determinants of a student's clerkship grade. In this chapter, we will discuss mistakes students commonly make on write-ups.

Mistake # 37

Not understanding the importance of the write-up

During the Internal Medicine clerkship, you will be expected to turn in write-ups on patients that you admit into the hospital. In most cases, it is the attending physician who will review them. At some schools, the clerkship director may also review one or two of your write-ups. Write-ups should not be taken lightly since the quality of the write-ups plays a large role in the determination of your overall grade.

Success tip # 28

Take great care in preparing your write-ups because the quality of your write-ups plays a large role in the determination of your overall grade

---

Mistake # 38

The write-up is not turned in on time

Write-ups should be turned in on time. Your evaluation may suffer if they are submitted late. Turning the write-up in on time also offers you another advantage. The attending physician may be able to return it to you before the next patient write-up is due. The feedback that you receive will help you prepare for the next write-up.

Success tip # 29

By turning write-ups in on time, the attending physician may be able to give you feedback before the next one is due.

Mistake # 39

The write-up is not complete

Patient write-ups done during the Internal Medicine clerkship are usually expected to be complete. This is in contrast to what you may have been asked to do during other rotations.

Success tip # 30

Students are expected to perform thorough and complete patient evaluations. Your write-ups should reflect the thoroughness of your evaluation.

Mistakes # **40** and # **41**

Not knowing what to include in the write-up
Not being familiar with the order of the write-up

What you include and how you present the information in the write-up may vary to some extent depending upon the preferences of your clerkship director or attending physician. At the beginning of the rotation, find out what you need to include by talking with the attending physician, clerkship director, and resident. If you do not have these conversations, you will see a lot of red marks on your write-ups when they are returned to you. Of course, red marks cannot completely be avoided on your first write-ups but by having these conversations, you will have fewer of them.

In general, the content of the write-up will be divided among the following elements:

- Chief complaint
- History of present illness (HPI)
- Past medical history (PMH)
- Past surgical history (PSH)
- Medications
- Medication allergies
- Social history
- Family history
- Review of systems (ROS)
- Physical exam
- Laboratory data
- Other studies (e.g., EKG, chest radiograph)
- Summary
- Problem list
- Assessment
- Plan

The previous list is also the order in which most attending physicians prefer the information presented. Write-ups that do not adhere to the expected order are considered disorganized and difficult to follow.

Success tip # 31

The savvy student recognizes the importance of asking the attending physician about any preferences he or she may have for the patient write-up.

Success tip # 32

For every patient, use the same format or order when presenting information in the write-up. The order should suit your attending physician's preferences.

Mistake # 42

The write-up does not include the date and time of the patient assessment

The date and time of your patient assessment should be at the top of every write-up. This sounds simple enough, but you would be surprised how often this information is not included.

Mistake # 43

Chief complaint or reason for admission is not listed

History taking begins with elicitation of the patient's chief complaint. When you ask the patient, "What brought you into the hospital today?" it is the patient's answer or description of the symptom that is the chief complaint. It is this answer that should be recorded as the chief complaint in the write-up.

Sometimes patients will answer this question with a medical diagnosis rather than a complaint. For example, the patient may say "kidney stones." If a diagnosis is offered rather than a description of a symptom, ask the patient to describe what it is that happened to prompt them to seek medical care. This will usually lead the patient to describe the symptoms experienced. This can be considered the chief complaint.

An exception to this rule occurs when a patient is transferred from another hospital for further care. In these circumstances, the patient does not have a new chief complaint and his or her last chief complaint (at the time of admission to the other hospital) has already been addressed. Here, the chief complaint can simply be the reason for the transfer. For example, if a patient is being transferred for further work-up of an unresolving pneumonia, you can say "reason for transfer is further evaluation of unresolving pneumonia."

You must also remember to convey to the attending physician a chief complaint that reflects the reason for the patient's hospital admission. It is not unusual for patients to complain of something which they feel is the reason for the hospitalization when in reality they are admitted for something entirely different.

Although the reason for the patient's hospital admission is usually stated in the patient's own words, there are times when this is not possible (e.g., comatose patient).

The chief complaint should be clearly stated in one sentence. Many attending physicians prefer to have the *duration* of the chief complaint included as well.

Mistake # <u>44</u>

The source of the history is not included

It is important to include the source of the history. In most cases, you will obtain information directly from the patient. At times, however, the source may be someone other than the patient (e.g., family member or friend). An example would be a comatose patient. In addition to indicating who provided you with the information, you should also comment on the reliability of the source.

> *Example:*
>
> *Information obtained from a clear and coherent patient.*

> *Example:*
>
> *Information obtained from a confused patient and his friend who brought him to the hospital. Old medical records were also used.*

Mistake # 45

The first sentence of the history of present illness (HPI) does not include the necessary information

Most attending physicians agree that the first sentence of the HPI should include the patient's age, sex, chief complaint, and duration of the chief complaint. Some also prefer to have the patient's race included in this opening statement while others only recommend doing so if it is relevant to their chief complaint. Marital status and occupation may also be included, again depending upon their relevance. If the patient has a history of a major medical illness that has bearing on the patient's reason for hospital admission, it too should be mentioned in the opening statement of the HPI.

> *Example:*
>
> *Mrs. Smith is a 64-year old Hispanic female with coronary artery disease, diabetes mellitus, and hypertension who presents with chest pain that lasted one hour in duration.*

37

Mrs. Smith may also have a PMH significant for sensorineural hearing loss but since this does not have direct relevance to her chief complaint of chest pain, it is not included in the opening statement of the HPI.

Mistake # **46**

The history of present illness (HPI) is not presented chronologically

The HPI is essentially a description of the patient's chief complaint. The HPI is the patient's story regarding the problem that prompted them to seek medical attention. It is universally considered to be the one of the most important elements of the patient write-up. The information conveyed provides key information for the diagnosis and management of the patient's illness.

The information in the HPI should flow like a story. After reading the HPI, the attending physician should have a clear idea of the events that transpired before the patient sought medical attention. Very few things irritate attending physicians more than a disjointed HPI, especially one in which the information is not presented chronologically.

An orderly story can usually be obtained by determining when the patient was last in his or her baseline or usual state of health. From there, the patient can repeatedly be asked, "What happened next?" until the story reaches the point of hospital admission. Along the way, clarifying questions about the patient's symptoms can be asked.

An example of how a chronological HPI may be written:

> *Example:*
>
> *Mrs. Smith is a 64-year old Hispanic female with coronary artery disease, diabetes mellitus, and hypertension who presents with chest pain that lasted one hour in duration. Patient was in her usual state of health until 3 days prior to admission when she first …Two days prior to admission….*

Mistake # 47

Not knowing what to include in the body of the HPI

Within the body of the HPI, you should include the following information:

- Description of the current complaint in detail (location, quality or character, frequency, onset, course, duration, severity, radiation [of pain], precipitating factors, alleviating factors)

- Associated symptoms

- Pertinent positives and negatives

- Description of how the symptom has affected the patient and his or her life (physically, emotionally, social relationships, others)

- What the patient thinks is wrong or has caused the problem

- What concerns the patient has

- Why the patient has sought medical attention now rather than earlier

Remember to also include information from the past medical history, family history, social history, and review of systems that is directly related to the current problem.

Mistake # **48**

The last sentence of the HPI is not worded properly

The HPI should end with the patient presenting to the emergency room or hospital. Your last sentence should often end with:

> *Example:*
>
> *… and so he came to the ER for evaluation.*

Mistake # **49**

Drawing conclusions or making judgments in the HPI

Refrain from drawing any conclusions or making any judgments in the HPI. For example, you may write, "the patient had shortness of breath and wheezing," but do not write, "the patient had symptoms consistent with emphysema."

Success tip # 34

Do not draw any conclusions from the HPI. Simply tell the patient's story.

Mistake # **50**

HPI is not written in full prose

In contrast to many of the other sections of the write-up, the HPI should be written in complete sentences. Short phrases or incomplete sentences should be avoided in this section.

Mistake # 51

Not knowing where to include the emergency room information

Most patients who are hospitalized are first seen in the emergency room. Before you and your team evaluate the patient, the ER physician will have performed a history and physical examination. Lab and other diagnostic tests may have been ordered. Some treatment may have also been administered.

A common question that students have is where they should place the ER information in the write-up. Should it be placed in the HPI or before the assessment and plan? There is no universal agreement on this issue and students should ask the attending physician about his or her preferences. Note that in mistake # 48, we recommended that the HPI should often end with the patient presenting to the ER. You may have to disregard this recommendation if your attending physician prefers to have the ER information included in the HPI. When reporting the ER information, do not list the impression or diagnosis of the ER physician. Instead, include only the facts.

Success tip # 35

Attending physicians differ on where, in the write-up, they would like the ER information to be included. Ask your attending physician about his or her preferences.

Mistake # 52

The past medical history (PMH) is not complete

The past medical history is really a list of the patient's medical problems. If the problems are related to the patient's chief complaint, they should also be reported in the first line of the HPI (see Mistake # 45). For each condition in the PMH, you should include the following information:

- When was the problem diagnosed?

- How was the problem diagnosed?

- What diagnostic studies (lab tests, radiologic studies, stress tests, pulmonary function tests, etc.) have been done? And if they have been done, what are the results?

- Dates of any surgeries for the problem

- Dates of any hospitalizations for the problem

- Therapy previously received

- Current therapy

- Current status of the problem

  Example:

  Hyperlipidemia: dx'd 1999, on simvastatin since then, reportedly with good control. Last lipids (7/00): Total chol - 155, LDL - 95, HDL - 30, Trig - 150

You may also include psychiatric, obstetric/gynecologic, and surgical problems here although some attending physicians prefer to list this information separately under the past psychiatric history, past obstetric/gynecologic, and past surgical history. Although medications, allergies, past hospitalizations, and significant childhood illnesses may be listed as part of the PMH, sometimes they stand alone in the write-up. Once again, ask the attending physician about his or her preferences.

Mistake # 53

Medication list is not complete

Under the heading, "medications," list all medications the patient is taking at the time of admission (outpatient medications), including over-the-counter and herbal medications. If the patient is not taking any over-the-counter or herbal medications, you should state so. Patients often forget or are reluctant to mention that they are on the following types of medications:

- Pain medicine

- Medicines for sleep

- Medicines for bowels

- Vitamins/minerals

- Birth control pills

- Skin creams

Students are recommended to specifically ask about each of these types of medications. If the patient is not taking any of them, state so in the medication section of the write-up.

Mistake # 54

Inpatient medications are included

Medications started since admission (inpatient medications) should not be listed under the heading, "medications," in the patient write-up. An exception to this rule is in the patient transferred to your team from another hospital service (e.g., intensive care unit or surgical service) or another hospital, in which case you should list the medications the patient was taking at the time of transfer.

Success tip # 36

When listing the patient's medications, do not include the medications you and your team started after the patient was hospitalized (inpatient medications). Include only the medications the patient was taking before the hospitalization (outpatient medications).

Mistake # 55

Medications are not listed by their generic names

Medications should be listed by their generic names. Some attending physicians, however, consider it acceptable to list medications by their brand names. It is best to ask your attending physician if he or she prefers the use of generic names.

Mistake # 56

Dosage, route, or frequency of the medication is not listed

Next to each medication, you should list the dosage, route, and frequency of the medication. If the dosage of the medication has been changed recently, it should be indicated. If the patient has been prescribed a medication but is not taking it, it is appropriate to list the medication here followed by the statement not taking in parentheses.

Example:

Enteric-coated aspirin 325 mg po qd
Metoprolol 50 mg po bid

*Felodipine 10 mg po qd (increased from 5 mg one
week ago)
Simvastatin 40 mg po qhs
Metformin 500 mg po bid (not taking)
Not taking any vitamins, minerals, or medicines for
sleep, bowels, or pain
No other over-the-counter or herbal medications*

Some attending physicians may prefer that you include the
indication (condition being treated) for the medication next to the
medication name.

Mistake # <u>57</u>

Patient's medication allergy is
not described

Under the heading, "allergies," list all of the patient's medication
allergies. The type of allergic reaction is often omitted but is of
major importance. In many cases, what a patient considers an
allergic reaction to a medication is actually a side effect of the
medication (i.e., nausea with codeine).

Example:

*Codeine - itching
Penicillin - rash and low blood pressure*

Other types of allergies (e.g., seasonal, contact) should not be
listed here but in the past medical history. If the patient does not
have any medication allergies, you can simply write "NKDA"
which is an acronym for "no known drug allergies."

Mistake # <u>58</u>

The social history is not complete

The social history provides information about the patient as a
person. It often includes information about the following:

- Marital status

- Number of children

- Occupation (current and previous, any toxic exposures)

- Living situation

- Personal interests/hobbies

- Smoking (can be listed under habits in the PMH as well)

- Alcohol use (can be listed under habits in the PMH as well)

- Recreational drug use (can be listed under habits in the PMH as well)

- Sexual history

It is also important to note that any social history relevant to the HPI should also be included in the HPI.

Success tip # 37

Any social history obtained that is relevant to the chief complaint and HPI should be included in the HPI.

Example:

Patient lives in Galveston with his wife and one son. He has worked as a construction worker for many years. He reports no known occupational exposures to asbestos or other hazardous/toxic chemicals. He has never been incarcerated. He has not traveled outside of southeast Texas for the past five years. He owns no pets. His relationships with his family, coworkers, and bosses are good.
Tobacco – 1 ppd X 25 years*
Alcohol – 3 beers/weekend
Recreational drug use – none currently or in the past
Tattoos – none
Transfusions - none
Sexual history – heterosexual, no contact with prostitutes, no history of homosexual contact

*Note that "ppd" refers to packs per day. The smoking history can also be reported in pack-years (pack-years = ppd X years smoked).

Mistake # 59

The family history is not complete

Some attending physicians ask their students to draw a family tree or pedigree, incorporating any illnesses that the members may have. Others simply want their students to make a list of close family members (parents, grandparents, siblings, children) along with any medical problems they have. No matter what your attending physician's preferences are, make sure that the family history is complete. It is also important to note that any family history relevant to the HPI should also be included in the HPI.

Success tip # 38

Any family history obtained that is relevant to the chief complaint and HPI should be included in the HPI.

Mistake # 60

The review of systems (ROS) is not thorough

The review of systems is an important part of the medical history. It is essentially a checklist of questions that should be asked just before the physical examination. The goal of these questions is to identify any significant symptoms that have not been elicited up until this point. A thorough review of systems may uncover important information. If you are having difficulty constructing a complete ROS, a useful resource is your physical diagnosis book.

If significant symptoms are uncovered in the review of systems, you should ask yourself if they are directly related to the patient's chief complaint and HPI. If so, then they should be included in the HPI. There is no need to repeat this information in the ROS. If the information is unrelated to the chief complaint and HPI, list it in the ROS under the appropriate heading. An example of an abbreviated ROS:

> *General:*
>
> *See HPI*
>
> *Head:*
>
> *See HPI*
>
> *Eyes:*
>
> *No blurring, pain, flashes, floaters, discharge, or double vision*
>
> *Ears:*
>
> *No pain, tinnitus, discharge, or hearing loss*

Of course, this is just an abbreviated ROS, one that doesn't include other important parts of the ROS like pulmonary, cardiovascular, gastrointestinal, etc. Note that you can simply state "see HPI" if the information has already been stated there.

Success tip # 39

Any review of systems information obtained that is relevant to the chief complaint and HPI should be included in the HPI.

Mistake # 61

The physical examination is not complete

Attending physicians expect medical students to perform complete physical examinations. Although residents and interns often perform more focused exams, it is your responsibility to be thorough and complete. This is because you are developing your physical examination skills at this point in your career. So even if you think that an ophthalmoscopic exam is not pertinent to your patient's chief complaint, it behooves you to perform this part of the physical exam. In the write-up, the complete physical examination should be documented.

Success tip # 40

The physical examination portion of the write-up should be thorough. Remember that residents and interns often perform and record focused physical exams but students are required to perform complete exams. Your write-up should reflect the completeness of your exam.

Guidelines for the physical exam section of the write-up

- Be complete
- Be specific
- If parts of the exam are omitted or deferred, be sure to indicate so
- Do not use nonspecific terms such as "negative," "normal," or "unremarkable"
- If necessary, draw a picture or diagram to describe findings

---

Mistake # 62

No comment is made about the patient's general appearance

Within seconds of meeting a patient, the experienced clinician can learn a lot by simply noting the patient's general appearance. Medical students often omit this in patient write-ups.

Mistake # **63**

Vital signs are not listed

Attending physicians expect medical students to take the patient's vital signs. They do not feel that it is appropriate to merely record the nurse's vital signs. Attending physicians want to make sure their students are comfortable with all aspects of the physical examination, including the taking of the patient's vital signs. In addition, if you report the nurse's vital signs, it does not really reflect your encounter with the patient. Forgetting to list the vital signs is a commonly made mistake on write-ups. Vital signs should be listed before the rest of the physical examination.

Success tip # 41

Omitting or forgetting to list the patient's vital signs is one of the most common mistakes students make on write-ups.

Mistake # **64**

Vital signs are listed as "afebrile and stable"

It is not appropriate to simply write that the "patient is afebrile with stable vital signs." The attending physician expects to see the actual numbers. Even normal values are helpful in supporting or arguing against the various considerations in the differential diagnosis of the patient's chief complaint.

Success tip # 42

Vital signs should not be recorded as "afebrile, vital signs stable" unless you are instructed to do so by the attending physician. Instead, include the actual numbers.

Mistake # 65

Orthostatic vital signs are omitted

It is not necessary to obtain and record orthostatic vital signs in all patients. When the patient presents with a disorder of volume or of the autonomic nervous system, however, orthostatic measurements of the blood pressure and pulse should be performed and reported. Medical students often forget to perform orthostatic vital signs or if performed, they often forget to record their findings.

Mistake # 66

Making judgments about the physical exam findings

When listing physical exam findings, simply report but do not make any judgments. Not uncommonly, students will report a finding and then state what they think that it is due to. For example, a student may write "irregularly, irregular rhythm noted due to atrial fibrillation." In this statement, "due to atrial fibrillation" should not have been included because it is not a physical exam finding but an assessment or judgment. During this part of the write-up, you must refrain from drawing conclusions about any physical exam findings.

Success tip # 43

Do not draw any conclusions about any physical exam findings in the physical examination section of the write-up. Simply report the findings.

Mistake # 67

Lab test results are not reported

All current laboratory test results (along with the date and time of the test) should be included in the patient's write-up, even if the values are normal. Previous lab test results should also be included if they have bearing on the patient's current clinical presentation. Circling the abnormal results is helpful to those reading your write-up.

Although lab test results may simply be listed one after another, some attending physicians prefer to have their students use stick figures to convey the information. Three stick figures that are commonly used include the following:

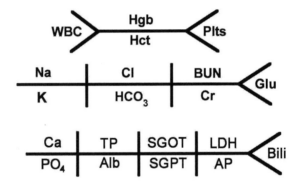

Mistake # 68

Basic lab test results are not reported first

List the results of the basic lab tests first. Basic lab tests include the complete blood count, coagulation tests (PT, PTT), basic chemistry profile (chem-7, electrolyte panel), and liver function tests (AST, ALT, alkaline phosphatase, albumin, bilirubin). Other blood test results can then be reported. After all blood test results are listed, report the results of the urinalysis, if performed.

Mistake # 69

Results of other studies are not reported

The results of other diagnostic studies should also be included in the write-up. These usually follow the laboratory data. These studies may include EKG, radiographs, other imaging tests, pulmonary function tests, etc. At times, the official report of these studies may not be available at the time the write-up is due. In these cases, offer your own interpretation and indicate that the official or final report is pending.

Mistake # 70

Summary is not included

After reporting the history, physical exam, and results of laboratory/diagnostic studies, a summary of the patient's clinical presentation should be included. This summary statement should be placed just before the problem list, assessment, and plan.

In the summary statement, summarize the important aspects of the patient's clinical presentation. Include significant aspects of the history, physical examination, and laboratory/diagnostic test results. The development of the summary is an exercise that requires you to focus on the most pertinent data in the patient's clinical presentation. It should not exceed 4 to 5 sentences in length.

Example:

In summary, Mrs. Smith is a 65-year old female with history significant for congestive heart failure who presents with complaints of 3 days of shortness of breath, orthopnea, paroxysmal nocturnal dyspnea, and leg swelling, which began after she ran out of her furosemide. Her physical exam is remarkable for distended jugular veins, S3, bibasilar crackles, and bilateral lower extremity pitting edema. Labs,

*including creatine kinase and troponin levels, and
EKG reveal no evidence of an ischemic event or
arrhythmia. Chest radiograph is notable for
cardiomegaly and pulmonary vascular redistribution.
Her clinical presentation is consistent with
exacerbation of congestive heart failure due to
noncompliance with medical therapy.*

Mistake # 71

Problem list is not complete

After the summary statement, a problem list should be included.
The problem list should be comprehensive. All significant
problems or abnormalities identified in the database (history,
physical exam, laboratory findings, etc.) should be included.
Initially, your problem list may be quite long but as you gain
experience in synthesizing data from the history, physical exam,
and laboratory data, you will be able to recognize relationships
between some of the problems. This will allow you to place them
under one heading rather than multiple headings. Most important,
early in your career, is the ability to identify all abnormalities.

Mistake # 72

Problem list is not prioritized

It is rare to have a patient with only one problem. When multiple
problems are present, it is important to prioritize the problems
identified. The presenting or primary problem should always be
listed first. The other problems should be listed in descending
order of importance.

Success tip # 44

***Problems in the problem list should be listed in
descending order of importance.***

Mistake # 73

Problems in the problem list are not as specific as possible

When listing problems in the problem list, it is important to be as specific as possible. For example, a patient may present with a chief complaint of chest pain. After consideration of the patient's history, physical examination, laboratory data, and other diagnostic test results, your diagnosis may be unstable angina. In this case, Problem # 1 on the problem list would be unstable angina rather than chest pain.

If the available evidence does not allow you to diagnose a specific disease, it is acceptable to be more general. In these cases, the problem may simply be reported as an unexplained symptom, sign, or test result. For example, if the etiology of the patient's chest pain is unclear after consideration of the history, physical examination, laboratory data, and other diagnostic test results, then Problem # 1 can be listed as chest pain.

Mistake # 74

The assessment is not included

You must make an assessment for every problem on the problem list. This involves carefully considering the clinical significance of each problem. If the etiology of the problem is not clear, then you must come up with a list of diagnostic possibilities. Once you have come up with this list, follow the steps in this box to construct the assessment.

Developing an assessment for problems of unclear etiology

Step 1: State the most likely diagnoses that can account for the problem.

> *Example: Although the differential diagnosis of problem X is long, the most likely possibilities include A, B, C, and D.*

Step 2: State the diagnosis that is most likely along with the key elements of the history, physical exam, and laboratory/ diagnostic data that supports it

> *Example: Of these possibilities, A is most likely because the patient has …*

Step 3: Discuss the other diagnostic possibilities and why they are less likely. If you can exclude one or more of these conditions, state so and provide support for these conclusions.

> *Example: B is less likely because the patient …*
> *C can be excluded because …*

When constructing the assessment, resist the temptation to simply copy information from a text. Instead, apply the information you learn from your reading to the patient's problems.

For problems of known etiology, the assessment does not need to be as extensive. For example, if the patient has a known history of hypercholesterolemia but is hospitalized for an entirely different reason, it is not necessary to develop an extensive assessment of hypercholesterolemia. Instead, it is sufficient to develop an assessment that includes the current status of the problem.

Example:

Hypercholesterolemia – Last LDL (performed one month ago) was 90, which is well within the target range for this patient with coronary artery disease.

56

Success tip # 45

Forgetting to include an assessment (for every problem!) is one of the most common mistakes students make. Review each problem to make sure you have not skipped the assessment.

Mistake # <u>75</u>

The plan is not included

A plan should follow an assessment for every problem in the problem list. The plan for the primary problem (Problem # 1 and other very active problems) should be detailed. Since many students find it particularly challenging to develop a plan for problems of unclear etiology, we have included the following box, which provides a strategy to help overcome this challenge.

Developing a plan for problems of unclear etiology

Step 1: List further diagnostic studies needed to confirm your working (most likely) diagnosis

Step 2: List further diagnostic studies needed to exclude other conditions in your differential diagnosis

Step 3: List treatment and management regimen for the problem

---

The plan is most often reported as a list. For example, in a patient diagnosed with pneumonia, the plan may be as follows:

> *Example:*
>
> *1. Sputum Gram stain and cultures (sent)*
> *2. Blood cultures (sent)*
> *3. Oxygen by nasal cannula at 2 liters/minute*
> *4. Intravenous gatifloxacin*

For a problem of known etiology that is not the reason for hospital admission, you can often skip over Steps 1-2 in the above box and move directly to Step 3. For inactive problems, it is acceptable to be brief.

Please note that some attending physicians prefer to separate the assessment section from the plan altogether while others recommend having the plan immediately follow the assessment of each problem. It is best to ask your attending physician about his or her preferences.

Success tip # 46

You may be required to include a discussion in your write-up that follows the assessment and plan. In the discussion, you may be free to expound upon a particular aspect of the patient's illness. For example, you may wish to discuss any new and recent changes in the evaluation or management of the patient's disease (do not forget to include references!). Even if you are not required to include a discussion, consider including one at the end of your write-up. Not only does it show initiative and desire to further your education but it also shows that you have read extensively about your patient's problem, all of which may impress the attending.

Presenting Newly Admitted Patients

For newly admitted patients, you will be expected to present the case during attending rounds on the day following the patient's admission into the hospital. The term "present" means to tell someone about a case, usually in a formal manner. The purpose of these oral case presentations is to inform the attending physician of the patient's illness. One of the major differences between the oral case presentation and the patient write-up is that the former must be succinct, without any unnecessary details. Attending physicians also rely on your case presentation to learn about your data collection and clinical reasoning process.

Since oral presentation skills are essential in facilitating the communication of patient information between healthcare professionals, much emphasis is placed on helping students acquire and develop effective oral presentation skills. Because oral case presentations have a significant impact on your clerkship grade, many students consider them to be one of the most stressful activities during the rotation. In this chapter, we will discuss common mistakes students make during oral case presentations on newly admitted patients.

Note: Readers should understand that there is some duplication of material between this chapter and the last chapter (commonly made mistakes on write-ups). This is done not only to stress the importance of these mistakes (many of which are crucial) but also to emphasize that it is common for students to avoid a mistake on the write-up only to make the same mistake on the oral case presentation. In the mistakes that these two chapters share in common, please note that the information in the body of the mistake may differ.

Mistake # 76

Not understanding the importance of the oral case presentation

The oral case presentation helps the attending physician get a good feel for what is going on with the patient. A solid presentation allows the attending physician to formulate a diagnostic and therapeutic plan. In addition, the quality of your oral case presentations plays a major role in the determination of your clerkship grade. One of the keys to impressing your attending physician is to deliver outstanding oral patient presentations on newly admitted patients.

Success tip # 47

Consistently delivering polished oral patient presentations on newly admitted patients is one of the keys to securing an outstanding evaluation.

Mistake # 77

Not realizing the type of presentation the attending physician is looking for

The type of presentation expected depends upon whether the patient is newly admitted or not. On post-call days, you will formally present your newly admitted patient to the attending physician. The attending physician expects a complete presentation because he or she is not familiar with the case. If the attending physician is familiar with the case (i.e. an old or established patient), a complete presentation is not necessary. Instead, you can give the attending a quick update on the patient's progress. Please refer to appendix A for more information on presenting old or established patients to the attending physician. The remainder of this chapter focuses exclusively on the presentation of newly admitted patients.

Mistake # 78

Not knowing how much time you have to present the case

The duration of the oral case presentation varies depending upon the preferences of the attending physician but is typically about 10 minutes. At the beginning of the rotation, you should ask the attending physician how much time you have to give your oral presentation on newly admitted patients. Remember that your attending has a preconceived notion as to how much time your oral patient presentation should take. He or she may not volunteer this information so it is a good idea to ask early in the rotation.

Success tip # 48

Early in the rotation, be sure to ask your attending physician how much time you have to give the oral patient presentation.

Mistake # 79

Oral case presentation goes beyond the allotted time

It is easy for oral case presentations to go beyond the time that is allotted for them. If you were to include every piece of information that you obtained during your patient encounter, the presentation would easily stretch beyond the allotted time. When oral case presentations last longer than expected, they take time away from other activities that need to be done during attending rounds. Usually, your team will have admitted other patients, all of which need to be discussed within the time designated for attending rounds.

If your attending physician prefers that the oral case presentation last no longer than 10 minutes, it is in your best interests to adhere to this rule. This, of course, requires you to time your presentation before delivering it to the attending.

Success tip # 49

Time your oral patient presentation while practicing. Do not exceed the time that has been given to you by your attending physician.

Mistake # **80**

Oral case presentation has too little or too much detail

How detailed an oral case presentation should be varies depending upon the preferences of the attending physician. Most internal medicine attending physicians expect detailed presentations, especially when compared to other rotations.

Before listening to your presentation, the attending physician has a preconceived idea as to the amount of information he or she wants to hear. Your goal is to avoid delivering oral case presentations that are too detailed or that are not detailed enough. The former tends to be more of a problem than the latter. Successful students must communicate an organized, succinct history, physical exam, assessment, and plan without losing the attending physician's attention. This can be a challenge, considering that there is so much material to convey on any given patient. It is no surprise that students commonly make the mistake of presenting too much information to the attending physician. Students who do not fall into the trap of "over-speaking" cases sound impressive to the attending physician because they are presenting at an above average level for their training.

How do you know what the attending physician wants? You can learn about the attending physician's preferences by meeting early in the rotation to discuss his or her expectations. Once you know exactly what the attending physician prefers, you can tailor the oral case presentation to meet his or her needs.

Success tip # 50

Delivering an oral case presentation with just the right amount of detail requires you to know the attending physician's expectations. If the attending physician is not available, ask the resident for guidance.

Mistake # **81**

Oral case presentation is a verbatim reading of the patient's write-up

The oral case presentation should not be a verbatim reading of the patient's write-up. Instead, it should be a carefully edited version of the write-up. That is because the oral and written case presentations have different purposes. The latter is much more comprehensive while the goal of the former is to rapidly convey key information regarding the patient's clinical presentation to the attending physician and other listeners. For this reason, the oral case presentation is less detailed than the write-up.

Success tip # 51

During your presentation, do not read your history & physical write-up verbatim. This is a sure way to annoy your team members (who are tired and post-call) and bore your attending physician. As a student, you must understand that your history/physical write-up is not the same as your oral case presentation. Your write-up always has more detail and information than your presentations. Your presentations should convey the big picture in the shortest amount of words possible.

Success tip # 52

When attending physicians assess the quality of your oral case presentation, they are not just interested in the content of your presentation but also in the way you come across. A presentation given in a monotonous voice with periodic mumbling will not impress anyone, even if you are right on target with the information you are conveying. That is why it is important to speak clearly and confidently with enthusiasm.

Mistake # 82

Oral case presentation is read

Students often wonder if it is permissible to use notes when giving their oral case presentations. This is a question that is best answered by the attending physician since preferences regarding the use of notes vary from one attending physician to another. In general, early in the rotation, greater reliance on notes is acceptable since unfamiliarity and discomfort with the oral case presentation is likely. As the comfort level increases, students become less reliant on their notes. Of course, when reporting medication dosages and laboratory data, it is necessary to refer to your notes so that the proper numbers and values are conveyed.

Less reliance on notes allows you to maintain eye contact with your listeners, which helps keep your audience interested in what you are saying. It also conveys to the attending physician that you have a firm grasp on your patient's clinical presentation and medical problems. If you are able to deliver polished oral case presentations without using too many notes, your efforts will be rewarded on your clerkship evaluation form.

Success tip # 53

Attending physicians are impressed with students who are able to deliver oral case presentations with a paucity of notes. The less notes you use, the better you will be regarded. It shows your listeners that you have command over the information.

Mistake # <u>83</u>

Not practicing your oral case presentation with your resident or intern

Be sure to practice your oral case presentation with your resident or intern before giving it to your attending physician. After your practice run, the resident or intern may offer you tips and suggestions to polish the presentation. Since residents are well versed in the art of delivering oral case presentations to attending physicians, their advice should be taken seriously. They can easily elevate the quality of your oral case presentation to a level beyond that of the average medical student.

Mistake # <u>84</u>

Not paying close attention to how the resident and intern present patients

Listen carefully to how your resident presents patients to the attending physician. Understand that most residents are veterans in giving concise, but informative, presentations. Simply observing them can be quite useful to you as you polish your own oral case presentation skills. Although it may be tempting, do not simply adopt their style of presentation because your attending physician will likely have different standards for oral case presentations given by students.

Mistake # 85

Letting the awkwardness and discomfort of the first few oral case presentations get to you

Even with considerable preparation, students often feel awkward and uncomfortable with their first few oral case presentations. These are natural feelings, which will abate with practice, time, familiarity with the oral case presentation, and an understanding of the attending physician's preferences. With time, your oral case presentations will become more polished.

Success tip # 54

Do not be concerned if your first few oral case presentations seem awkward. With practice, you will feel more confident.

Even though some early awkwardness is inevitable for most students, the key to starting off on the right foot with your first oral case presentation is adequate preparation.

Success tip # 55

Remember that you do not have a second chance to make a successful first impression. Prepare well, and try your best to give a very good first presentation to your attending. It is better to start at the top than at the bottom.

Mistake # 86

The information is not presented in the proper order

Present the patient information in the following order:

- Chief complaint
- History of present illness (HPI)

- Past medical history (PMH)
- Medications
- Medication allergies
- Social history
- Family history
- Review of systems (ROS)
- Physical exam
- Laboratory data
- Other studies (e.g., EKG, chest radiograph)
- Summary
- Assessment
- Plan

Oral case presentations that do not adhere to the expected order are considered disorganized and difficult to follow. Please note that the order is the same for both the write-up and oral case presentation.

Note: While most attending physicians prefer to have the review of systems presented just before the physical exam, some ask their students to present the information right after the history of present illness.

Mistake # **87**

Patient is not adequately identified

Before presenting the patient's chief complaint, it is important to provide the attending physician with the following information:

- Patient's name
- Patient's room number
- Patient's medical record number

This sounds simple enough but you would be surprised at how often students omit this information and begin with the chief complaint, only to have the attending physician interrupt them for the name and location of the patient.

Success tip # 56

Consider giving your attending physician a label with the patient's name and medical record number stamped on it. These labels are usually available at the nursing units. Ask the unit clerk for one.

Mistake # 88

Chief complaint or reason for admission is not expressed in the patient's own words

History taking begins with elicitation of the patient's chief complaint. When you ask the patient, "What brought you into the hospital today?" it is the patient's answer or description of the symptom that is the chief complaint. Many attending physicians feel that it is this answer that should be conveyed to the team as the chief complaint during the oral case presentation. The chief complaint should be clearly stated in one sentence. Many attending physicians prefer to have the duration of the chief complaint included as well.

Be sure you link the chief complaint with the reason for admission. For example, if the patient has a severe pneumonia, but comes in complaining about his skin rash, do not put "skin rash" as your chief complaint. The reason you are admitting this patient is for his severe pneumonia and not for the skin rash. The diagnosis that you want the listener to derive from your presentation is the pneumonia and not the skin rash. Since the chief complaint should be a symptom and not a diagnosis, it also would not be acceptable to list pneumonia as the chief complaint. Instead, one or more of the symptoms that the patient has (which are due to pneumonia), should be listed as the chief complaint. Again, the chief complaint should be a symptom and not a diagnosis.

An exception to this rule occurs when a patient is transferred from another hospital for further care. In these circumstances, the patient does not have a new chief complaint and his or her last chief complaint (at the time of admission to the other hospital) has already been addressed. Here, the chief complaint can simply be the reason for the transfer. For example, if a patient is being transferred for further work-up of an unresolving pneumonia, you can say "reason for transfer is further evaluation of unresolving pneumonia."

Mistake # 89

The source of the history is not included

After providing the patient's name, room number, medical record number, and chief complaint, you should inform listeners of the source of the history. In most cases, the history will be taken directly from the patient. At times, however, the patient may be unable to provide the history. In these cases, information may be obtained from family members or friends. You should also indicate the reliability of the informant (i.e., person providing the history).

Mistake # 90

The first sentence of the history of present illness (HPI) does not include the necessary information

Most attending physicians agree that the first sentence of the HPI should include the patient's age, sex, chief complaint, and duration of the chief complaint. Some also prefer to have the patient's race included in this opening statement while others only recommend doing so if it is relevant to their chief complaint. Marital status and occupation may also be included, again depending upon their relevance. If the patient has a history of a major medical illness that has bearing on the patient's reason for hospital admission, it too should be mentioned in the opening statement of the HPI. An example:

> *Example:*

> *Mrs. Smith is a 64-year old Hispanic female with coronary artery disease, diabetes mellitus, and hypertension who presents with chest pain that lasted one hour in duration.*

Mrs. Smith may also have a PMH significant for sensorineural hearing loss but since this does not have direct relevance to her chief complaint of chest pain, it is not included in the opening statement of the HPI. If the patient has no significant PMH, indicate that in the opening statement.

> *Example:*

> *Mrs. Smith is a 64-year old Hispanic female with no significant PMH who presents with chest pain that lasted one hour in duration.*

Notice also that the patient's name is used in the opening statement rather than the words, "This is a 64-year-old Hispanic female…." Using the patient's name shows the listener that you consider the patient a person and is more respectful.

Mistake # 91

The history of present illness is not presented chronologically

The HPI is essentially a description of the patient's chief complaint. The HPI is the patient's story regarding the problem that prompted them to seek medical attention. It is universally considered to be the one of the most important elements of the oral case presentation. The information conveyed provides key information for the diagnosis and management of the patient's illness.

The information in the HPI should flow like a story. After listening to the HPI, the attending physician should have a clear idea of the events that transpired before the patient sought medical attention, starting from the time the patient was last at baseline (i.e., usual state of health). Very few things irritate attending physicians more than a disjointed HPI, especially one in which the information is not presented chronologically.

An orderly story can usually be obtained by determining when the patient was last in his or her baseline or usual state of health. From there, the patient can repeatedly be asked "What happened next?" until the story reaches the point of hospital admission. Along the way, clarifying questions about the patient's symptoms can be asked.

An example of how a chronological HPI may be presented is as follows:

Example:

Mr. Jones is a 53-year old male with poorly controlled diabetes mellitus who presents with a two-day history of fever, flank pain, and dysuria. Patient was in his usual state of health until two days prior to admission when he developed … One day prior to admission, he …

Success tip # 57

It is said that 80 to 90% of diagnoses are made from a good history and physical exam. Your attending physician is relying on the information you provide in the HPI to make a diagnosis. That is one of the reasons why it is so important to make sure the HPI is chronological.

71

Success tip # 58

Try your best to present the HPI chronologically. It is annoying and difficult for the attending to follow a story that jumps from one occurrence to another without chronology. This forces the attending physician to stop the presentation and ask you questions in order to reconfirm the sequence of events. This wastes time.

Mistake # 92

Not knowing what to include in the body of the HPI

Within the body of the HPI, you should include the following information:

- Description of the current complaint in detail (location, quality or character, frequency, onset, course, duration, severity, radiation [of pain], precipitating factors, alleviating factors)

- Associated symptoms

- Pertinent positives and negatives

- Description of how the symptom has affected the patient and his or her life (physically, emotionally, social relationships, others)

- What the patient thinks is wrong or has caused the problem

- What concerns the patient has

- Why the patient has sought medical attention now rather than earlier

- Information from the past medical history, social history, family history, and review of systems that is directly related to the patient's chief complaint should also be included here.

Mistake # 93

The last sentence of the history of present illness is not worded properly

The HPI should end with the patient presenting to the emergency room or hospital. Your last sentence should often end with:

> *Example:*
>
> *... and so he came to the ER for evaluation.*

Mistake # 94

Not knowing where to put the ER information

Most patients who are hospitalized are first seen in the emergency room. Before you and your team evaluate the patient, the ER physician will have performed a history and physical examination. Lab and other diagnostic tests may have been ordered. Some treatment may have also been administered.

Students are often unclear about when to discuss ER information in their oral case presentations. Should it be discussed in the HPI or later in the presentation? There is no universal agreement on this issue and students should ask the attending physician about his or her preferences. Note that in mistake # 93, we recommended that the HPI should often end with the patient presenting to the ER. You may have to disregard this recommendation if your attending physician prefers to have the ER information included in the HPI. When reporting the ER information, do not mention the impression or diagnosis of the ER physician. Instead, include only the facts.

Success tip # 59

Before your first oral case presentation, be sure to ask the attending physician about when he or she would like to hear about the ER information.

Mistake # 95

Too much time is spent on the past medical history (PMH)

The past medical history is really a list of the patient's medical problems. If the problems are related to the patient's chief complaint, they should also be included in the first line of the HPI (see mistake # 90). The past medical history that you obtain from the patient should be a detailed account of all past and present medical problems. Information about psychiatric disease, surgeries, obstetric/gynecologic conditions, injuries, accidents, and childhood illnesses may also be considered part of the past medical history.

In your write-up, the past medical history should be comprehensive but, because of time constraints, you must pare it down for the oral case presentation. This requires you to include only the most important information about major problems. This can be a challenge, especially if patients have a laundry list of medical problems. Here, you must choose which of the medical problems are significant enough for inclusion in your oral case presentation. To make this decision, you need to ask yourself if including the condition will help your attending physician better understand the patient's current clinical situation.

Mistake # 96

Medication list is not complete

It is important to obtain the patient's complete medication list. In some cases, doing so is quite easy because the patient will bring in a list of their medications. Remember to always ask about any over-the-counter or herbal medications since patients often do not consider them to be "medications." In particular, always ask specifically about medicine taken for pain, sleep, and bowels.

You will also encounter patients who have no clue as to what their medications are. They may start by telling you, "I take a green pill and two white pills." In these cases, you may have to call a family member for the medication history.

Success tip # 60

If you obtain the patient's medication list from the old medical records, be sure to review the list with the patient. Make sure that the patient is taking the medications. Since medication errors are quite common, it is best to be thorough here.

It is acceptable to discuss some of the patient's medications before the medication section of the oral case presentation if you feel the information has bearing on the patient's current illness. For example, if the patient has been noncompliant with heart failure medications and is now hospitalized with congestive heart failure exacerbation, it is certainly reasonable to mention this in the HPI.

Mistake # 97

Medications are not listed by their generic names

Medications should be reported using their generic names rather than trade names. Some attending physicians, however, consider it acceptable to use trade names.

Mistake # 98

Dosage, route, or frequency of the medication is not known

For some attending physicians, a simple list of the current medications without any information regarding dosage, route, or frequency of the medications is sufficient. Others expect their medical students to include this information. What you will include will vary with your attending physician's preferences. Irrespective of what your attending physician prefers, you need to have this information readily available in order to provide appropriate patient care.

Mistake # 99

Inpatient medications are included

Medications started since admission (inpatient medications) should not be reported when conveying the patient's medication list to the attending physician. Only the medications the patient was taking at home (outpatient medications) should be reported. An exception to this rule is in the patient transferred to your team from another hospital service (e.g., intensive care unit or surgical service) or another hospital, in which case the medications the patient was on at the time of transfer should be included.

Success tip # 61

When reporting the patient's medication list, only describe the medications the patient was taking before hospitalization (outpatient medications). Do not include medications started after the patient was hospitalized (inpatient medications).

Mistake # **100**

Not knowing details regarding the patient's medication allergies

If the patient reports being allergic to a certain medication, you must include the reaction the patient developed. Many patients believe they are allergic to a certain medication when, in fact, what they experienced was a medication side effect. One of the most common mistakes made is not eliciting the details of the reaction.

Mistake # **101**

Too much time is spent conveying the social history

Students are expected to take a complete social history. The bare necessity for all student-obtained social history should include smoking history (in pack years), alcohol history, recreational drug history (be sure to delineate IV drug use), history of promiscuity or incarceration, occupation, exposures, recent travel, marital status, and number of children. Also note the home situation. This is important for discharge planning. You certainly do not want to send patients, who are unable to care of themselves, home unless there is a family member or other caregiver capable of providing the necessary assistance. Generally, during oral case presentations, since we are most interested in the smoking, alcohol, and drug history, present this information first.

Example:

Patient has a 50 pack year smoking history and currently smokes 3 cigarettes per day. He has a history of alcohol abuse, but quit drinking 5 years ago. He smokes marijuana every so often, but denies any history of IV drug use. He claims to be monogamous. No history of incarceration. Works as

*a factory worker and reports history of exposure to
asbestos. He lives with his partner. No recent travel.*

It is best to be brief when conveying the social history unless it
has significant bearing on the patient's current illness. Social
history that is directly related to the patient's illness should be
included in the HPI.

Mistake # **102**

Too much time is spent conveying the family history

It is best to be brief when conveying the family history unless it
has significant bearing on the patient's current illness. Family
history that is directly related to the patient's illness should be
included in the HPI. If the family history is not important, you can
simply say that it was "noncontributory."

Mistake # **103**

Too much time is spent conveying the review of systems

The review of systems is essentially a series of questions that
should be asked of the patient just before the physical
examination. The goal of these questions is to identify any
symptoms that the patient may have experienced recently. The
review of systems should be complete. If you are having difficulty
constructing a complete ROS, a useful resource is your physical
diagnosis book.

When presenting the ROS, however, including everything would
make your presentation stretch on and on. Find out in advance
what your attending expects to hear in the ROS. Many attending
physicians prefer that their students convey only significant
symptoms, which are defined as ones that are important enough

to be included in the problem list. If there are none, you should simply say that the review of systems was noncontributory.

Success tip # 62

When you perform a history, be sure to obtain a complete review of systems. During the oral case presentation, you cannot convey the entire review of systems to your listeners. That alone would take up much of your allotted time. Instead, you must only include any symptoms you feel are significant.

Note: While most attending physicians prefer to have the review of systems presented just before the physical exam, some ask their students to present the information right after the history of present illness.

Note: Remember that information already discussed in the HPI does not need to be repeated here.

Mistake # 104

Review of systems duplicates information already conveyed in the history of present illness

Some of the elements of the review of systems may have already been discussed in the history of present illness. If so, there is no need to repeat this information. For example, in the patient presenting with chest pain, the patient's responses to questions asked in the cardiovascular review of systems should be included in the history of present illness. This is because the answers to these questions (pertinent positives and negatives) are directly relevant to the patient's chief complaint of chest pain. It is not necessary to repeat this information when conveying the review of systems information.

Mistake # **105**

Too much time is spent conveying the physical exam findings

Although you are expected to perform a complete physical examination, if you include everything in your oral case presentation, it alone would take up a considerable portion of your allotted time. For this reason, while all positive findings need to be conveyed, negative findings do not need to be mentioned unless they have bearing on the patient's clinical presentation. Some attending physicians, however, prefer to hear about the heart, lung, and abdominal exam in every patient, even if the findings are negative. Again, discussion with your attending physician early in the rotation will shed light on his or her preferences.

Success tip # 63

While you are expected to perform a thorough history and physical examination, you cannot report the entire exam to your listeners during the oral case presentation. It simply takes too much time. That is why most attending physicians like to hear only about pertinent aspects of the exam.

Mistake # **106**

Not following the appropriate order

The order in which physical exam findings are presented varies from clinician to clinician. It is best to ask your attending physician early in the rotation about any preferences he or she may have. Here is one order that you can use:

- General appearance
- Vital signs

- HEENT

- Neck

- Chest

- Cardiovascular

- Abdomen

- Genitourinary/rectal/pelvic

- Extremities

- Neuro

- Musculoskeletal

- Skin

Mistake # 107

No comment is made about the patient's general appearance

Within seconds of meeting a patient, the experienced clinician can learn a lot by simply noting the patient's general appearance. Medical students often omit this in their oral patient presentations.

Mistake # 108

Vital signs are not mentioned

Forgetting to mention the vital signs is one of the most common mistakes students make. Quite often, students have the vital signs but for some reason, skip over it. In other cases, the information was not written on the note card the student is using to present the case. When the attending physician interrupts the presentation to ask for the vital signs, students often fumble around searching for the information. To avoid this from happening, always have the vital signs readily available.

Mistake # **109**

Medical student states that the patient is afebrile and vital signs are stable

It is not appropriate to simply say that the "patient is afebrile with stable vital signs." The attending physician expects to hear the actual numbers, irrespective of whether they are normal or abnormal.

Success tip # 64

When reporting the admission vital signs, do not say that the patient was "afebrile and vital signs were stable". Instead, provide the attending physician with the actual numbers. If the patient is noted to be volume depleted on admission, remember to mention orthostatic changes in the blood pressure and heart rate.

Mistake # **110**

Making judgments about the physical exam findings

When reporting physical exam findings, simply report but do not make any judgments. Not uncommonly, students will report a finding and then state what they think it is due to. For example, a student may say "costovertebral angle tenderness was noted due to pyelonephritis." In this statement, "due to pyelonephritis" should not have been included because it is not a physical exam finding but an assessment or judgment. You must refrain from drawing conclusions about any physical exam findings during this part of the oral case presentation.

Success tip # 65

When reporting the physical examination findings, refrain from drawing any conclusions regarding the findings. Simply report the findings.

Mistake # **111**

Lab test results are not reported

Some attending physicians may prefer that all of the patient's current laboratory test results be conveyed. Others require only pertinent positives and negatives. If you are not sure what the attending physician expects, it is best to present all the lab data, even if the results are normal. Although this sounds simple enough, you would be surprised at how often students do not have the laboratory test results readily available. You should also have results of previous lab test results in the event that the attending physician asks for them. Attending physicians almost always ask for previous test results when a patient presents with a low hemoglobin/hematocrit or high BUN or creatinine. In these cases, the previous test results provide information on what the patient's baseline values are.

Mistake # **112**

Basic lab test results are not reported first

Convey the results of the basic lab tests first. Basic lab tests include the complete blood count, coagulation tests (PT, PTT), basic chemistry profile (chem-7, electrolyte panel), and liver function tests (AST, ALT, alkaline phosphatase, albumin, bilirubin). Other blood test results can then be reported. After all blood test results are conveyed, report the results of the urinalysis, if performed. Quite often, students skip around. Skipping around is one sign of a disorganized oral case presentation.

Success tip # 66

Report the results of related tests together. For example, liver function test results should be reported together.

Mistake # **113**

Results of other studies are not reported

The results of other diagnostic studies should also be included in the oral case presentation. These should follow the laboratory data. These studies may include EKG, radiographs, other imaging tests, pulmonary function tests, etc. At times, the official report of these studies may not be available before delivering the oral case presentation. In these cases, you should offer your own interpretation and indicate that the official or final report is pending. It is important to bring the study to rounds so that your attending physician can review it while you are describing the findings.

Success tip # 67

After presenting the lab values, show the attending physician any available studies including EKGs, chest films, or CT scans. Be prepared to interpret these studies. But very often the attending physician will ask another medical student on the team to read the EKG, for instance, because he or she is not familiar with the study compared to the student presenting the case.

Success tip # 68

Do not forget to bring the EKG and chest film to attending rounds. This requires you to gather these studies beforehand. Do not forget to bring old studies for comparison.

Mistake # <u>114</u>

Summary is not brief

Following the reporting of the laboratory and diagnostic test data, your listeners will be ready for your summary. There are many ways to present the summary section. One commonly preferred method is to present a very brief summary, describing the patient's medical problems along with the reason for hospitalization or diagnosis. Unlike the summary in the write-up section (see Mistake # 70), here it is generally shorter, usually no longer than 1-2 sentences.

> *Example:*
>
> *Mr. Smith is a 63-year old black male with diabetes mellitus, hypertension, and congestive heart failure who presented to us last night with CHF exacerbation.*

Mistake # <u>115</u>

Plan is discussed before assessment

The assessment and plan come right after your summary statement. It is the most important part of the oral case presentation because it is the only part that highlights your thought processes and ideas. If it is done well consistently, the attending physician will be impressed with the quality of your oral case presentation. Since it is the last part of the oral case presentation, what you say here and how you say it will be the final impression you leave the attending physician with.

The assessment and plan is a troublesome area for many students and many crucial errors can be made here. Chief among these is skipping the assessment completely and moving directly to the plan. Before discussing diagnostic testing and therapeutic measures that you and the team have recommended, provide an assessment of the problem. An example of an assessment followed by a plan:

> *Example:*
>
> *Problem #1. CHF exacerbation. This is suggested by his symptoms of orthopnea and paroxysmal nocturnal dyspnea and by the signs of bilateral crackles on lung exam, elevated JVP and the lower extremity swelling. We will check an echo to assess the cardiac function. We will salt restrict his diet, start him on IV lasix at 40 mg every 12 hours, and we will monitor his progress by measuring his daily weight.*
>
> *Problem #2…*

Here is an example of bypassing the assessment and going straight to the plan. This is to be avoided.

> *Example:*
>
> *Problem #1. CHF exacerbation—we will check an echo and start the patient on IV lasix, salt restricted diet, and we will weigh the patient daily.*

If the diagnosis is not conclusive by the available evidence, you should include a differential diagnosis in your assessment. For example, if the patient is being admitted for shortness of breath from a possible pulmonary embolism, you can present the assessment and plan as follows:

> *Example:*
>
> *Problem #1. Shortness of breath. Possible etiologies include CHF exacerbation, COPD exacerbation and pneumonia. However, given the acute onset of pleuritic chest pain and the right leg deep vein thrombosis diagnosed by the ultrasound, we believe the shortness of breath is likely due to a pulmonary embolism. Result of the CT chest with PE protocol is pending. We have already started the patient on Lovenox.*

Since patients usually present with multiple problems, you will discuss the assessment and plan for each problem. Be sure to discuss problems in descending order of importance. Be sure to address every issue that is pertinent to the patient's care. Do not forget to discuss the social issues, especially if they are relevant to the patient's disposition.

Note: Some attending physicians may prefer you to use a systems-based rather than problem-based approach for presenting the assessment and plan. If this is the case, please refer to mistake # 129 for more information.

Mistake # 116

Not seeking feedback about your oral case presentations

Midway through the rotation, ask the attending physician for constructive criticism in regards to your performance during the rotation, particularly on your oral case presentations. This will help you improve your performance and grade.

The Daily Progress Note

You will be expected to write a daily progress note for every patient you are following. You are "following" a patient if you are participating in his or her care. The purpose of the daily progress note is to update readers of the patient's hospital course since the last progress note was written. Other health care professionals rely heavily on the daily progress note, especially the assessment and plan, to learn not only about the patient's progress but also about the current diagnostic and therapeutic plan. In this chapter, mistakes students commonly make on the daily progress note are discussed.

Mistake # 117

Not reviewing how to write the progress note with the intern or resident at the beginning of the rotation

At the start of the rotation, be sure to meet with the resident or intern to discuss how the daily progress note should be written. This is especially important if the Internal Medicine clerkship is your first rotation, in which case you may be unsure of how to start. More seasoned students will still benefit from this type of meeting because daily progress notes do differ from one rotation to another. In addition, residents and interns may have their own preferences, which they will want to share with you.

Mistake # 118

Not writing legibly

All of your efforts to write a good progress note will be for naught if your writing is not legible. If readers of the medical record cannot read your handwriting, you might as well not write the note at all because the information you are conveying is not accessible. Take the time to write as legibly as you can.

Mistake # **119**

Not listing the date and time of the note

The date and time of the note are essential for legal purposes. In addition, readers of the medical record will be better able to understand the order in which things have happened in the patient's hospital course. Forgetting to date and time the progress note is one of the most common mistakes students make.

Mistake # **120**

Not identifying the type of note you are writing

The title of the note must always be included. The title should indicate your level of training as well as the type of note you are writing.

Example: M3 Progress Note

Mistake # **121**

Not following the proper order

Daily progress notes should be written using the SOAP format. SOAP is an acronym for "subjective, objective, assessment, and plan." In the subjective portion of the note, the patient's complaints are listed. In the objective section, the physical exam and laboratory data are reported. The note concludes with your assessment and plan.

Order of the daily progress note

Date and time of the progress note
Title
Level of training
Type of note being written
Subjective statement
Medication list
Physical examination
Laboratory/diagnostic test results
Assessment and plan
Signature

You will encounter departures from the SOAP format, especially when you read notes written by senior clinicians. Refrain from adopting these different styles unless the resident, intern, or attending physician instructs you to do so.

Mistake # **122**

Not knowing what to include in the subjective statement

The subjective statement is essentially the patient's assessment of his or her condition. Write down all of the patient's events and complaints over the last 24 hours. For example, if the patient was hospitalized for abdominal pain, you should comment on whether it is still present and, if so, how it has changed. You should also comment on any pertinent positives and negatives (for abdominal pain, comment on nausea, vomiting, diarrhea, constipation, etc.). Also report any new complaints that have developed.

Mistake # **123**

Not including the medication list

Students are often asked to list all active medications after the subjective statement. Some residents or attending physicians may prefer that the active medication list be written in the left or right margin of the daily progress note. Inclusion of the patient's medication list helps others to immediately see what medications the patient is taking. Mention the medication name, dose, route, and frequency (e.g. Gatifloxacin 400 mg IV qd). If the patient is taking an antibiotic, indicate how many days they have been on it (e.g., Gatifloxacin 400 mg IV qd [Day # 4]).

Mistake # **124**

Not including the general appearance of the patient

Always start your physical exam section of the daily progress note with a comment about the patient's general appearance.

Mistake # **125**

Not including the vital signs

After recording the patient's general appearance, list the vital signs, including temperature (current and maximum [Tmax]), heart rate, respiratory rate, blood pressure, and pulse oximetry (oxygen saturation) readings (also include amount of oxygen being given). If the vital sign values are fluctuating in a patient, it is a good idea to give ranges of these values over the last 24 hours. After reporting the vital signs, list the 24-hour intake and output (I&O), daily weight, IV fluid rates, and other objective values (i.e., accuchecks) that may pertain to the patient.

Students often forget to record the vital signs. Others have a tendency to write "patient afebrile, vital signs stable" rather than the actual values. Unless instructed to do so by your resident, intern, or attending physician, always include the actual values.

Success tip # 69
Vital signs should be listed. Avoid writing "patient afebrile, vital signs stable" unless asked to do so. Don't forget to include trends, if needed.

Mistake # 126

Physical examination is not focused

Unlike your admission history and physical or write-up, the physical exam recorded in the daily progress note should be brief and focused. You are not required to include a complete physical examination. Instead, the focus should be on parts of the physical exam that are relevant to the patient's current complaints or illness.

For example, if the patient is presenting with cellulitis of the right arm, it is important to describe the physical exam findings of the arm. Although you may have palpated his spleen when the patient was first admitted into the hospital, there is no need to examine the spleen or record exam findings related to the spleen again because the information is not relevant to the patient's illness.

Most attending physicians, however, do recommend a basic examination of the heart, lungs, abdomen, and extremities in every patient on a daily basis. These findings should be reported in the physical exam.

Mistake # 127

Not including the results of laboratory and diagnostic studies

Following the physical examination section of the daily progress note, the results of laboratory and diagnostic studies should be written (along with the date and time of the test). Start with lab test results. Here, it is not necessary to include the results of all tests done since the patient was admitted. Instead, record the lab test results that have returned since the previous day's progress note. If lab test results are pending at the time the note is written, indicate that the test result is pending. If the results return later in the day, the information can be charted in the form of an addendum.

After recording lab test results, list the results of any other diagnostic testing. When listing the results of radiologic studies, indicate whether the results are preliminary or final.

Mistake # <u>128</u>

Assessment and plan are not properly done

Most clinicians prefer the assessment and plan to be written in problem list format. In this format, the patient's medical problems are listed in descending order of importance. For example, a patient who is hospitalized with a COPD exacerbation, may also have a history of hypertension and gout. During the hospitalization, the patient is noted to be hypertensive but the gout is under control. For this patient the problem list would be as follows:

1. COPD exacerbation
2. Hypertension
3. Gout

COPD exacerbation would be problem # 1 because it is the most important problem, the one that prompted the hospitalization. Problem # 2 would be hypertension because the patient's blood pressure is not well controlled. Gout would be listed last because it is currently under control.

When listing problems, remember to be as specific as possible. For example, a patient with COPD exacerbation often presents with shortness of breath. If the patient's clinical presentation is consistent with COPD exacerbation, then Problem # 1 should be COPD exacerbation. If, however, the etiology of the shortness of breath is not clear, then it is appropriate to list Problem # 1 as shortness of breath.

Next to each problem, offer an assessment or current status of the problem. Too often, students forget to include the assessment and move directly to the plan.

> *Example of an assessment: 2. Hypertension - Blood pressure not well controlled with systolic values ranging from 150 to 170.*

Following the assessment, document the plan. The plan may consist of further diagnostic testing and/or changes in management.

> *Example of an assessment and plan: 2. Hypertension - Blood pressure not well controlled with systolic values ranging from 150 to 170. Will increase metoprolol from 25 to 50 mg po bid and continue hydrochlorothiazide at the same dose.*

Mistake # 129

Not knowing whether to use a problem-based or systems-based approach to present the assessment and plan

In Mistake # 128, we described a problem-based format for presenting the assessment and plan. An alternative format is the systems-based approach, which is quite commonly used in the intensive care unit. Some clinicians prefer to use it in non-ICU patients as well but many prefer the problem-based format rather than the systems-based approach. Be sure to ask your intern, resident, or attending physician whether you should use the problem-based or systems-based approach when documenting the assessment and plan.

Success tip # 70

The important thing to remember, regardless of which method used, is to be clear and concise, yet to not leave out significant information.

In the systems-based approach, each problem is a system. An example:

1. Pulmonary

2. Gastrointestinal

3. Cardiovascular

While some prefer to list the systems in a particular order irrespective of the patient's primary problem, others list the systems in descending order of importance.

Next to each system relevant issues are discussed. For example, if the patient is hospitalized with acute cholecystitis, the assessment and plan may be listed as follows:

1. Gastrointestinal - Acute cholecystitis - symptoms and signs improved. Continue NPO, intravenous antibiotics, and intravenous fluids.

When using the systems-based approach, there is often a tendency to omit the name of the condition or problem the patient has. An example:

1. Gastrointestinal - Unchanged. Continue NPO, intravenous antibiotics, and intravenous fluids.

In the above example, the name of the problem being treated was omitted. Readers of the note would not know why the patient is being treated with antibiotics and fluids.

Some important points about the assessment and plan

Wait until work or attending rounds have been completed before writing your final plan when possible.

Never write something you are unsure of.

If for some reason you disagree with the resident or intern, do not put it on paper.

Spend time on the assessment and plan. Put considerable thought into this section. Residents and attending physicians read your assessment and plan in order to gauge your understanding of the patient's problems.

Mistake # **130**

Forgetting to sign your name

Do not forget to sign your signature at the end of every progress note. Forgetting to do so is one of the most common mistakes students make. Underneath your signature, print your name, level of training, and beeper number legibly. It is important to have your intern, resident, or attending physician cosign your note before you place the note in the patient's chart.

Mistake # **131**

Scribbling out errors in the progress note

Because the patient's hospital chart is a legal document, mistakes made on the progress note should not be scribbled out to the point that the error is no longer legible. Instead, you must cross it out with a single horizontal line. After crossing out the error, label it as an "error." Then initial and date it. When mistakes are not handled in this fashion, it may raise suspicion that someone was trying to hide something.

Mistake # **132**

Not seeking feedback on the quality of your progress notes

In a perfect world, your intern, resident, or attending physician would review the progress note with you. We can tell you that this often does not happen. Quite often, progress notes written by students are simply cosigned without any feedback being given regarding the quality of the notes. Do not be afraid to seek feedback if you find yourself in this type of situation.

Success tip # 71

Be proactive in seeking feedback on the quality of your progress notes. Too often, attending physicians and residents do not take the time to review progress notes with their students.

Mistake # 133

Delaying the writing of the progress note

It's often in your best interest to write the note early in the day. After all, you never know when the patient (and his or her chart) may be taken off the floor for tests or procedures, some of which may take a long time to perform. Quite often, students delay writing the progress note because they want to wait for the results of tests, which often return later in the day. But there is no need to wait because these test results can be charted later in the form of an addendum. Another reason to write notes early is that your note needs to be reviewed and cosigned by the intern or resident. You certainly don't want to run into the situation where the intern or resident, having completed all of their work, are simply waiting for you to finish your note so that they can go home.

Your progress notes also provide useful information that residents and interns can review, such as medications, labs, and study results. Getting your notes in the charts early will save them time from looking up all the information. Finally, your progress note may contain important points that residents and interns may not know, so it is very helpful to complete note writing early in the day.

Success tip # 72

Make it a goal to complete your progress note early in the day. If necessary, additional information can be charted later in the form of an addendum.

> *Example: Addendum - Pulmonary consultant called. They have evaluated the patient and plan to perform bronchoscopy this evening.*

Attending Rounds

The attending physician is the most senior member of the team. In addition to making sure that patients assigned to the team receive the best possible care, he or she is also responsible for teaching the house officers and medical students on the team. Your interaction with the attending physician will mainly occur during attending rounds, a period of time during which the entire team typically meets. What occurs during attending rounds will vary from day to day. If your team admitted patients the day before, the attending physician will expect to hear about these new patients. Typically, the most junior member of the team, who is following the patient, will present newly admitted patients to the attending physician. If there are no new patients to present, the attending physician may ask for updates on previously admitted patients, discuss interesting aspects of patients' illnesses, conduct bedside rounds, or have team members give talks. Although teaching styles differ, many attending physicians like to ask students questions, especially about diseases your patients have. In this chapter, we will discuss common mistakes students make during attending rounds.

Mistake # <u>134</u>

Not knowing how to present patients to the attending physician

In the first few days of the clerkship, you must determine how your attending physician would like you to present patients. You can learn about the attending physician's preferences by meeting with him or her early in the rotation. If the attending physician is not available to you, your intern or resident can fill you in. As a general rule, there are two types of oral case presentations:

- Presentation of newly admitted patients

- Presentation of established patients (i.e., patients your attending physician is familiar with)

Mistakes students commonly make when presenting newly admitted patients have already been discussed in Part V of this book. For previously admitted or established patients (patients that the attending physician is already familiar with), provide a quick update on the patient's hospital course (what has happened since the last time you discussed the patient with the attending physician). Simply present the patient to the attending like you did during that day's work rounds (see Part II) with the resident and intern (keep it brief and to the point!). Be sure to include any recommendations and revisions made by your resident during work rounds. For more information on presenting old or established patients, please refer to Appendix A.

Success tip # 73

Remember to ask your attending at the beginning of the month about his/her expectations of you during the rotation. Find out how he or she wants you to present patients and what to include in your patient write-ups. At mid-month during the rotation ask your attending about your performance and if there are any areas that need improvement.

Mistake # 135

Differential diagnosis of the patient's chief complaint is not known

A patient's chief complaint is usually a symptom that prompted them to seek medical care. Every symptom has its own differential diagnosis. The term "differential diagnosis" refers to a list of conditions that could account for the patient's symptom. It is common for attending physicians to ask their students for the differential diagnosis of the symptom that led to the patient's hospitalization.

For example, if the patient is hospitalized with chest pain, you should know the differential diagnosis of chest pain. For many symptoms, the differential diagnosis can be quite extensive. It is not necessary to memorize and regurgitate all of the possibilities. Instead, you should focus on the more common causes of the patient's symptom. In addition, life-threatening etiologies should always be considered. Do not be surprised if the attending physician asks you what the life-threatening causes of the patient's symptom(s) are.

If asked to provide a differential diagnosis for a symptom, you can say:

> *Although there are many causes of symptom X, we should consider the more common and life-threatening etiologies such as …(5-10 conditions is a reasonable list).*

Success tip # 74

The successful medical student is able to demonstrate to the attending physician his or her understanding of the patient's chief complaint and the approach to the complaint's work-up. For example, if your patient's chief complaint is shortness of breath, you should know the different causes of this symptom, and how you rule in or out these causes through history, physical, and diagnostic studies.

Mistake # 136

Not having a differential diagnosis for a sign

Physical exam findings, signs, or abnormalities may either be related to the patient's chief complaint or symptoms or be unrelated to the patient's current illness. Every physical exam finding has its own differential diagnosis. It is common for attending physicians to ask their students for the differential diagnosis of physical exam findings such as jaundice, abdominal distention, peripheral lymphadenopathy, and lower extremity edema.

When a finding is noted, look over your differential diagnosis for the patient's symptom and use the step by step approach in the following box to prepare for your attending physician's questions.

Preparing for the Attending Physician's Questions about Physical Exam Findings, Abnormal Lab Test Results, and Imaging Test Findings

Step 1: Look up and be familiar with the differential diagnosis of every physical exam finding, abnormal lab test result, or imaging test abnormality

Attending physicians commonly ask students for the differential diagnosis of physical exam findings, abnormal lab test results, and imaging test abnormalities.

Step 2: Determine if the physical exam finding, abnormal lab test result, or imaging test abnormality supports any of the conditions in the differential diagnosis of your patient's symptom

Attending physicians want to know if you are able to link the physical exam finding, abnormal lab test result, or imaging test finding with one of the conditions in the differential diagnosis of the patient's chief complaint.

Step 3: If the physical exam finding, abnormal lab test result, or imaging test abnormality is not supportive of any of the conditions in the differential diagnosis, consider the possibility that it is unrelated to the patient's current illness

Step 4: If it is unrelated to the patient's current illness, develop an approach to determining the etiology

Physical exam findings, abnormal lab test results, and imaging test abnormalities that are unrelated to the patient's current illness may still be important and require evaluation. This step will help you prepare for the question, "What work-up should we do to determine the etiology of this finding or abnormality?"

Mistake # 137

Differential diagnosis of an abnormal lab test result is not known

It has become standard practice to obtain basic laboratory tests in every hospitalized patient. Other tests may also be ordered, depending upon your patient's illness. Although an occasional patient may have completely normal laboratory test results, most have one or more lab test abnormalities. It is important to not only make note of these abnormalities but also to develop a differential diagnosis for each. Every abnormal lab test result has its own differential diagnosis. Again, it is common for attending physicians to ask their students for the differential diagnosis of abnormal lab test results. Follow the step by step approach in the box on 101 to prepare for your attending physician's questions.

Success tip # 75

Abnormal lab test results commonly encountered during the clerkship include low hemoglobin/hematocrit (anemia), low platelet count (thrombocytopenia), low sodium (hyponatremia), metabolic acidosis, and abnormal liver function tests (AST, ALT, alkaline phosphatase, bilirubin, albumin). Be prepared to provide the attending physician with the differential diagnosis and approach to determining the etiology of the abnormality.

Mistake # 138

Clinical significance of an imaging test abnormality is not understood

Imaging test abnormalities may either be related or unrelated to the patient's current illness. Every imaging test abnormality has its own differential diagnosis. As is the case with physical exam findings and abnormal lab test results, be prepared to give a differential diagnosis of imaging test abnormalities. Follow the box on page 101 to prepare for your attending physician's questions on imaging test findings.

Mistake # **139**

Not being well read on your patient's primary problem

Many of the questions attending physicians like to ask students deal with different aspects of the patient's diagnosis. For example, if your patient has acute pancreatitis, you should be prepared to answer questions about the incidence, epidemiology, pathogenesis, risk factors, differential diagnosis, clinical features (symptoms and signs), laboratory studies, imaging/other diagnostic studies, prognosis, complications, and therapy of this condition.

For the patient's primary problem, be prepared to answer questions about the following:

Incidence

Epidemiology

Pathogenesis

Risk factors

Differential diagnosis

Clinical features (symptoms and signs)

Laboratory studies

Imaging/other diagnostic studies

Prognosis

Complications

Therapy

Although your attending physician is not likely to ask you about everything in the above box, reading about these aspects of the patient's illness will further your knowledge and help prepare you for the clerkship exam.

Success tip # 76

You should know as much about your patients and their problems as possible. Knowing about your patients' diseases will prepare you for the attending physician's questions. Attending physicians usually ask medical students high yield, basic medical questions. Your personal readings, as well as teaching during work rounds, can help you learn the answers to these questions. Try your best to answer, but don't worry! You are not expected to know everything. It's okay to say, "I don't know."

Mistake # **140**

Not being well read on the patient's other problems

Although patients may be hospitalized for one problem, keep in mind that they often have other problems. Too often, students focus entirely on the primary problem and ignore secondary problems. This often leaves students at a loss to answer questions attending physicians may ask about these problems.

In addition, reading about the patient's other problems will certainly help you if these problems become more active during the hospitalization. Let's take, for example, a patient hospitalized with acute pancreatitis due to alcohol use. The student who reads about acute pancreatitis and alcoholism rather than just acute pancreatitis alone will be in a better position to manage the patient. Should this patient develop alcohol withdrawal, the reading done will help the student recognize the manifestations, evaluation, and treatment of this condition. In addition, the knowledge gained will help the student answer the attending physician's questions.

Mistake # **141**

Indication for obtaining the chest x-ray is not known

There are many indications for ordering a chest radiograph. In the past, an admission chest radiograph was a routine part of the patient's initial work-up. Currently, however, many clinicians do not believe that the chest x-ray should be a standard part of the evaluation of every hospitalized patient. Instead, they recommend that the study be obtained if it is clinically indicated. You should not be surprised if your attending physician asks you why a chest film was performed. You should be ready with an answer. Also keep in mind that the same question may be asked of you with regards to other imaging tests (e.g., abdominal film).

Success tip # 77

Always understand the indications for ordering a laboratory or imaging test. Be ready to explain the reason to your attending physician, if asked.

Mistake # **142**

Chest film is not systematically interpreted

Experienced clinicians (like your attending physician) may be able to make radiologic diagnoses quickly, without the need for systematic inspection of the chest film. Very few medical students, however, can call themselves experienced when it comes to interpreting chest x-rays. For inexperienced clinicians, it is best to approach every chest film systematically. Be sure to develop a system in which every aspect of the film is scrutinized. This will ensure that important findings are not missed. If you have not been introduced to a system, check with your intern or resident, who will be happy to share their system with you. Remember to always follow the same sequence of analysis. One system that you may use is described in the following box.

Systematic Approach to Chest Film Interpretation (PA or AP film)

Patient name/number

Date of study

Comment on whether it is a PA or AP film

Comment on rotation of the patient

Comment on penetration of the film

Bones

Breasts

Soft tissue

Costophrenic angle

Lung markings/fields

Mediastinum

Cardiac shadow

Cardiac chambers

Comparison with previous chest film

Please refer to Appendix E for more information on chest film interpretation.

Mistake # 143

Chest film is not brought to rounds

If you are presenting the patient during attending rounds, be sure to bring the chest film (and other imaging studies) with you. Your attending physician will want to review it with you. It will save the team from having to make a trip to the radiology reading room. At most institutions, you will be able to check out the patient's imaging tests. Sometimes, copies of the films can be made and given to you for rounds.

Expect the attending physician to ask you to describe the chest film findings during your oral case presentation. Since you know this is likely to happen, prepare for it in advance by doing the following:

1. Interpret the film by yourself systematically

2. Review the film with your resident or intern. Ask them to comment on your interpretation.

3. Review the film with the radiologist (when time permits). Ask them to comment on your interpretation (see Mistake # 144).

If you follow these three steps, you are more likely to impress the attending physician with your chest film interpretation skills.

Mistake # <u>144</u>

Chest film is not reviewed with the radiologist

Whenever possible, review the chest film and other imaging studies with the radiologist. Do not just place the film in front of the radiologist and wait silently for his or her interpretation. Instead, offer the radiologist your own interpretation of the film. The radiologist will appreciate your efforts and he or she will be more inclined to educate you about the film. Always remember to provide the radiologist with the patient's clinical history and any specific questions you have. Imaging studies are best evaluated with the patient's clinical context in mind.

Too often students review the films only with the resident or intern. While the resident and intern are probably more experienced than you, they do not have the expertise of a radiologist.

Radiologists are often available to you at all hours of the day. At some institutions, however, radiologists or radiology residents may not be on site at all times, especially during the evening and nighttime hours. In these situations, you can still review the films with the radiologist, but you will probably have to wait until the morning. There will usually be time before attending rounds for you to make a trip to the radiology department. If you do not make this trip, you will lose a valuable educational opportunity.

In addition, discussion with the radiologist may very well prepare you for the attending physician's questions about the chest film.

Mistake # __145__

Not knowing how to interpret a chest film you have never seen

Attending physicians commonly ask students to interpret films they have never seen before. Quite often, these films are of patients that you are not following. It's easy to get flustered in these situations but a few simple techniques can help you regain your composure. Before saying anything, allow yourself 15 to 20 seconds to simply look at the film. If need be, you can buy yourself a little more time by asking one of the team members to give you a brief clinical description of the patient. After all, films are best interpreted when the interpreter has the patient's clinical situation in mind. After you have regained your composure and looked over the film, provide your thoughts. Once again, be systematic in your approach.

Mistake # __146__

EKG is not systematically interpreted

Most patients that are assigned to you will require an EKG. To avoid missing important findings, it is essential to analyze every EKG systematically. During your clerkship, you will see that your attending physician can often make rapid EKG diagnoses, without the need for systematic inspection of the tracing. With time and experience, you will become more adept at reading EKGs, which will decrease the time needed for interpretation. For now, however, it is best to approach every EKG systematically. If you have not been introduced to a system, check with your intern or resident, who will be happy to share their system with you. Remember to always follow the same sequence of analysis. One system that you may use is described in the following box.

> ## Systematic Approach to EKG Interpretation
>
> Rate
> Rhythm
> Intervals (PR, QRS, QT)
> Blocks
> Axis
> Hypertrophy
> Conduction disturbances
> Myocardial injury/infarction
> ST-segment changes
> T-wave changes
> Q waves
> Changes from previous EKG

Please refer to Appendix D for more information on EKG interpretation.

Mistake # <u>147</u>

EKG is not brought to rounds

If you are presenting the patient during attending rounds, be sure to bring the EKG with you. Your attending physician will want to review it with you. It will save the team from having to make a trip to the chart to find it later.

Expect the attending physician to ask you to describe the EKG findings during your oral case presentation. Since you know this is likely to happen, prepare for it in advance by doing the following:

1. Interpret the EKG by yourself systematically

2. Review the EKG with your resident or intern. Ask them to comment on your interpretation. The resident or intern will be able to point out any findings you may have missed.

This review will serve you well as you prepare for attending rounds.

3. Be sure you know the criteria for any abnormalities that are present (i.e., left bundle branch block) as well as the clinical significance of the findings.

If you follow these three steps, you are more likely to impress the attending physician with your EKG interpretation skills.

Mistake # **148**

Not knowing how to interpret an EKG you have never seen

Do not be surprised if the attending physician asks you to interpret an EKG that you have never seen before. Many students lose their composure when asked to interpret an EKG on the spot. To maintain your composure, just remember that you are not expected to be proficient with EKG interpretation. Although the attending physician knows that you may not have all the answers, he or she has asked you to interpret the EKG because it is only through time, experience, and practice that students become comfortable with EKG interpretation. When asked to interpret an EKG, allow yourself 15 to 20 seconds to simply look at the EKG. This pause will also help you regain your composure. If you need some more time, consider asking one of the team members to give you a brief clinical description of the patient. Then, go ahead and offer your thoughts. Once again, as with chest film interpretation, be systematic in your approach.

Mistake # **149**

Not bringing in an article

To further your team's knowledge, consider bringing in an article about your patient's illness. A recent review article on the condition can supplement what you and the team have already learned from your reading of the traditional textbooks. Keep in mind that textbooks quickly become outdated and, in many areas of medicine, advances occur at a remarkable pace. If questions that come up during rounds remain unanswered, take the initiative and perform a literature search. Share what you have found with the rest of the team at the appropriate time. Your attending physician, resident, and intern will be impressed with your initiative and appreciate your efforts to further their education. This will certainly help your clerkship evaluation—in fact, on some clerkship evaluation forms, evaluators are asked to comment on whether their students have performed literature searches.

Mistake # <u>150</u>

Not grading yourself after attending rounds

After every attending rounds, you should ask yourself the following questions:

- What did the attending physician ask me?

- Was I ready for the questions?

- How did I answer each question?

- Did any of the questions surprise me? If so, which ones?

- How can I use this experience to better prepare me for the next day's attending rounds?

This is one of the keys to identifying any areas that you need to brush up on. For example, let us say that the attending physician keeps asking you about how to work up abnormal lab test results and you haven't been able to answer the questions to your satisfaction. Once you have identified this to be a problem area, your next step is to figure out why it's a problem area. Are you not reading about lab tests? Do you not have the right resources to answer these questions? Once you have pinpointed why it's a problem, then you can take steps to prepare yourself better for attending rounds.

Success tip # 78

At mid-month during the rotation ask your attending about your performance and if there are any areas that need improvement. You may wish to ask the attending physician what he or she thinks about your work ethic, motivation, enthusiasm, organization, professionalism, fund of knowledge, problem-solving skills, and quality of your oral case presentations/write-ups. The attending physician will be asked to comment on these on your evaluation form.

Appendix A: Presenting Established Patients

Presenting patients who have been in the hospital for some time (established patients) differs from presenting patients who are newly admitted. Whereas the new patient presentation requires more details on all aspects of the history, physical, assessment, and plan, the oral presentation on an established patient focuses on providing an update on the patient's hospital course. The new patient presentation is discussed in Part V of this book. Here we will briefly discuss the presentation of established patients.

Always start with a one-line statement that includes the patient's name and why the patient is here. This reminds the listening audience of the patient you are presenting.

> *Example: Mr. Jones is a 55-year-old man with diabetes and a history of peptic ulcer disease who was admitted yesterday with melena.*

Then proceed with the rest of your presentation using the **SOAP** format. This stands for Subjective, Objective, Assessment and Plan.

S: Present all the "Subjective" data. A common preference is to start with how the patient is currently doing and then present a summary of events since you last discussed the patient. Some people include any new information or recommendations from consultants in this summary.

> *Example: The patient is currently doing well with no complaints. He denies any further episodes of melena. GI evaluated the patient yesterday and is planning to do an EGD this morning.*

O: Report all the "Objective" data. This includes the vital signs, the physical exam, and results of labs and studies.

First, present the vital signs, using numbers. Do not say, "Vital signs are stable." Do not forget to mention the blood glucose, daily weight, and oxygen saturation, if applicable. Also pay attention to trends, particularly in the vital signs and in the lab values.

Example: He has been afebrile with Tmax 99 and Tcurrent 98.6. His blood pressure is currently 140/80 with a pulse of 70. Respirations is 12. His blood glucose values have been 108, 115, and is 120 this morning.

Next, present the physical exam. You do not have to present a detailed and thorough physical exam over again (like the one you presented when the patient was first admitted into the hospital). Instead, you should present a focused physical exam, but always include the general appearance, heart, lung, abdomen, and extremity exam. If they are unremarkable and unchanged since admission, a common preference is to say that they are unchanged since admission. If there are remarkable findings, then make sure you describe them

Example:

On exam, the patient appears well, his heart, lung, and abdominal exams are unchanged since admission. He still has trace pre-tibial edema on his bilateral lower extremities and the left foot ulcer appears worse today. There is worsening erythema...etc.

When presenting labs, do not present old lab results unless they are pertinent. Present the latest lab results. This is another area where noting trends is very important. The attending physician and resident want to know how the pertinent lab values have changed. This information helps them understand if the condition or problem is improving or worsening. Also, report any new study results.

A/P: Present the assessment and plan of old patients by starting with a one line summary of the patient and why this person was admitted. Present the assessment and plan as described in the presenting new patient chapter; however, the emphasis now is on presenting follow up information and on the plan of action. Make sure you also address what is needed before the patient can be discharged home.

Success tips

- Avoid reading your notes during presentation of established patients

- For complicated and very ill patients, pay extra attention to details and be more thorough on your presentation, especially in the assessment and plan

- Practice your presentations with your colleague and with the resident or interns on the team

- Do not digress and talk about trivial matters. Stay focused.

Appendix B: Ward Etiquette

Understanding the proper "unwritten mannerisms" is very important to your success. Failure to recognize some of these etiquettes will be detrimental to your evaluations by the resident and attending.

- **Never be late.** Never have the team wait for you.

- **Never lie.** A more appropriate thing to say is "I'm sorry, I don't know, but I'll find out."

- **Be a team player.** Be helpful at all times, even if the work does not pertain to the patients you are following, i.e. getting xrays for another patient, etc.

- **Dress professionally.** Wear professional attire with a clean, pressed white medical student coat. Impressions are very important.

- **Be courteous to everyone.** Not only is this the right thing to do, but also you never know when you need help. Nurses, clerks, and other staff members can be very helpful. Also, sometimes their inputs to the resident and attending figure into your evaluation.

- **Do not show up any team member.** You would be surprised how often this happens.

- **Never forge signatures.** This still happens.

- **Be enthusiastic and attentive at all times,** even if the team is not discussing your patients.

- **Communicate with the team.** Always notify some member of the team, usually the resident, if you have to leave. A friendly "I'm leaving for lecture" will make a lot of difference to the resident. Always remind the team of any future absences.

- **Notify your team immediately if your patient is not doing well.**

- **Never tell patients information that you are not sure of.** Defer to your team.

- **Don't ever go home without being dismissed by the resident.**

- **Do not talk about patients in public places where there are other people** (e.g. elevators). This is a patient privacy act violation.

- **Remember to date and time every page of the admission H & P, progress notes, addendum, and orders. Be sure to have them cosigned by the resident or intern.**

Appendix C: TIPS (General Pearls)

Here are a few general tips that will help you become successful in your clerkship rotation.

- Prior to starting the rotation, ask other medical students who have done the rotation for some tips and advice.

- Make sure you have a pager before starting the rotation.

- Be organized with all your patient data and always be prepared to present and discuss your patients.

- See your patients more than once per day. Always check on your patients and review the patient charts and any new labs prior to going home.

- Whenever you give talks to the team about certain topics, make nice handouts.

- Understand that the input of the resident and intern have considerable impact on your attending's evaluation of you.

- Know your evaluation criteria. Here are some of them in no particular order of importance: personality (ability to work with others, interaction with staff), work ethic, write-ups, oral presentations, fund of knowledge, professionalism, initiative, motivation, problem-solving skills, organization, and bringing in literature.

- Make sure you have all the necessary tools for the rotation: stethoscope, alcohol wipes (to clean your equipment after each patient), penlight, tuning fork, visual acuity card, ophthalmoscope, etc.

- Familiarize yourself with the setting. Tour the nursing unit to see where the following things are located: medication administration record, portable blood pressure cuff, supply room, computers, chart rack, where forms are kept, and most importantly, where the bathrooms are located.

APPENDIX C: TIPS (GENERAL PEARLS)

- In addition, know the locations of the following places:

  - Emergency Room and General medicine clinics

  - Units: key nursing units, dialysis unit, intensive care units (MICU, CCU)

  - Radiology: Xrays, CT scans, and nuclear medicine

  - Laboratories: chemistry, microbiology, hematology, blood bank

  - Cafeteria

  - Medicine Office and conference rooms

- Check the patient's medication list daily. Sometimes medications get left off or dropped from the list. This happens more often than you would expect and is a common cause of medication errors.

- Have a pocket reference book or palm software readily available to look up information. There are many good ones. Ask other medical students what are the latest and most helpful ones.

- Read about your patients' problems and diagnoses. Familiarity with the disease processes may help with your presentations as well as help you come up with good, intelligible questions to ask.

- Take notes on teaching points made by residents and attendings on your patients as well as your co-students' patients. The chances that these teaching points will come up again in "pimping" questions are very high, even with the same attending and resident.

- Above all, be prompt, organized, concise, and prepared!

Appendix D: Basic EKG

Note: this section serves as a quick reference for common things noted on EKGs. It provides general concepts only. This section should not used as the sole resource for learning EKGs. You should read other books to understand the fundamentals of EKGs.

Start by looking at the EKG to see if there is anything that overtly presents itself and then proceed with a step-wise approach addressing each of the following: (Note: there are many approaches and we have provided one of them).

EKG Reading

Rate
Rhythm
Intervals
Blocks
Axis
Hypertrophy
Myocardial Injury/Infarction

Rate: Find an R wave (from QRS complex) that lands on a dark line. Start counting down each large box until you reach the next R wave. Say to yourself after each large box: 300-150-100-75-60-50. This will give you the approximate rate. If the complex falls between two lines, just estimate the rate between the two respective values. For severe bradycardia, count how many complexes you have on an EKG (generally this is a 6 second strip) and then multiply by 10.

What is the rate?

> Normal Heart Rate: 60-100
> Tachycardia: > 100
> Bradycardia: < 60

Rhythm: What is the patient's heart rate?

> Normal ⇨ Proceed to A
> Tachycardic ⇨ Proceed to B

A: Normal Heart Rate

Look at Lead II or V1. Is there a P wave before every QRS complex?*

Yes—Is the rhythm regular?

Regular ⇨ **Sinus Rhythm**

Irregular ⇨ What is the P wave morphology?

Same morphology ⇨ **Sinus Arrhythmia**

Different morphology ⇨ **Wandering Pacemaker**

* If you are unsure whether or not there is a P wave before every QRS because of artifacts on the EKG, see if the rhythm is regular or irregular. If it is irregular, it is most likely atrial fibrillation.

B: Tachycardias

Look at the QRS complexes. Are they wide or narrow (>100 ms or ½ large square)?

● Narrow complex ⇨ Is the rhythm regular or irregular?

Regular ⇨ What is the P wave morphology?

Upright P before QRS ⇨ **Sinus Tachycardia**
Atypical P before QRS ⇨ **Atrial Tachycardia**
Sawtooth Pattern ⇨ **Atrial Flutter** (with fixed block)
Retrograde P after QRS ⇨ **AVRT**
No P or Retrograde P distorting QRS ⇨ **AVNRT**

Irregular ⇨ What is the P wave morphology?

No P waves ⇨ **Afib with Rapid Ventricular Response**
3 or more different P waves ⇨ **Multifocal Atrial Tachycardia**
Sawtooth ⇨ **Arial Flutter** (with variable block)

● Wide complex ⇨

Ventricular Tachycardia
Supraventricular Tachycardia (any of the above tachycardias) **with Aberrancy,** such as a bundle branch block or accessory pathway

Intervals: Note the normal length of the following intervals:

PR	120-200 ms (3-5 small boxes)
QRS	< 100 ms (less than ½ of a big square)
QT	340-430 ms (less than ½ the distance between 2 R waves)

Further discussion of interval lengths is beyond the goal of this appendix.

Blocks: Note the following:

Look in V1: if there is a widened QRS (> 100 ms) and the complex points—

Down ⇨ then think of **LBBB (left bundle branch block)**

Up ⇨ then think of **RBBB (right bundle branch block)**

Atrial-Ventricular Blocks (AVB)

1st degree—The PR interval is >200 ms (one large square)

2nd degree—

MobitzType I (Wenckebach)—progressive prolongation of PR until there is a dropped QRS (a P wave without a QRS complex)

Mobitz Type II—regular and periodic dropped QRS

3rd degree (complete)—complete AV dissociation. P wave and QRS complex have independent rhythms

Axis: Normal axis is between -30 and +100. Greater than +100 is right axis deviation (RAD) whereas less than -30 is left axis deviation (LAD). Look at the QRS complex in leads I and aVF and see if it is pointing up or down. Remember the following:

Leads	Normal	LAD	RAD
I	∧	∧	∨
aVF	∧	∨	∧

Success Tip

Pretend that your left thumb is Lead I and your right thumb is Lead aVF. When both thumbs are up, then everything is normal. When the LEFT thumb is up and the right thumb is down, think LEFT axis deviation. When the RIGHT thumb is up and the left one is down, think RIGHT axis deviation. When both thumbs are down, then the axis is indeterminate.

Hypertrophy:

Remember: Atrium ⇨ look at P wave

Ventricle ⇨ look at QRS complex

Atrial Hypertrophy:

Is the P wave ≥ 1 mm in depth in Lead V1? ⇨ **Left Atrial Hypertrophy**

Is the P wave > 2.5 mm tall in Lead II? ⇨ **Right Atrial Hypertrophy**

Ventricular Hypertrophy: There are many criteria. Here are a few popular ones.

• S wave in (V1 or V2) + R wave in (V5 or V6) > 35 mm • R wave in aVL >12 mm • R wave in I > 14 mm	⇨ **Left Ventricular Hypertrophy**
• R/S ratio in Lead V1 > 1 • Right axis deviation	⇨ **Right Ventricular Hypertrophy**

Myocardial Injury/Infarction: The following information reflects generalities. There are many exceptions for which the explanations are beyond the scope of this appendix. Keep in mind the goal of this section is to teach basic EKG reading.

There are several major types of changes that signify myocardial injury or infarction. They are the following:

> *Q wave* = infarction (isolated q wave in Lead III is not significant)
>
> *ST segment elevation* = acute injury
>
> *ST depression* = subendocardial injury or infarction
>
> *T wave inversion* = ischemia

When looking for myocardial injury, one must look at contiguous leads and look for congruous changes. Contiguous leads are leads that depolarize towards similar axis. For example, leads I and aVL are both leads that depolarize from right to left, so they are considered contiguous. If changes are present only in one lead, then it is generally thought to be insignificant. The following are groups of contiguous leads and they describe the location of the ischemia or infarction:

> **I, aVL** - lateral
> **II, III, aVF** - inferior
> **V1-V2** - septal
> **V3-V4** - anterior
> **V5-V6** - lateral
> Tall R wave in **V1-2** - posterior MI

> You can put them together. For example, ST depressions in I, aVL, and V3-6 would be regarded as anterolateral ischemia.
>
> Also, any new LBBB is equivalent to an acute ST elevation MI.

Whenever you have changes in the inferior leads (II, III, aVF), get a "right-sided EKG." If there is ST segment elevation in RV4 (right-sided V4), then this is regarded as right-sided (right

ventricle) ischemia or infarction. Management would be different
from left-sided (left ventricle) disease. To obtain a right-sided
EKG, you would need to flip the precordial leads to the right side.

Miscellaneous:

1. **Hyperkalemia** – peak T waves ⇨ prolonged PR ⇨
   flattening of P wave ⇨ widening of the QRS

2. **Pericarditis** – diffuse ST elevations, PR interval
   depressions, T-wave inversions

3. **Pericardial Effusion** – electrical alternans, low voltage.

4. **Wolf-Parkinson -White** – short PR interval, delta wave,
   widened QRS (> 0.10 sec)

5. **Pulmonary Embolism** – most common EKG tracing is
   sinus tachycardia. Can also see the incomplete/complete
   RBBB and $S_I Q_{III} T_{III}$

Appendix E: Basic Chest X-Ray Interpretation

Note: the purpose of this section is to introduce an approach to reading chest x-rays. Do not use this as the only resource for learning chest radiology. Generalizations are made in this section to simplify the concepts. Words can never replace pictures, so make sure you go look at plenty of x-rays.

Identifier: You do not want to make management decisions based on wrong x-rays.

Check the patient name and medical record number

Check the date of the study

Is this a PA or AP film?

> *PA:*
>
> *Front side of the chest lies next to the film.*
> *Heart is minimally magnified and the heart borders are sharp.*
>
> *AP:*
>
> *Back is lying next to the film.*
> *Heart is magnified with fuzzy borders.*

Is this film rotated?

Unrotated film ⇨distance from the sternum to each end of the clavicle should be equal.

What is the penetration of the film?

If the film is *too white* and you cannot see the spine behind the heart ⇨ **underexposed**

If the film is *too black* and you cannot see the vessels of the lung ⇨ **overexposed**

How do I approach reading the rest of the film?

There are many approaches to reading the chest film. One approach is to start from the center of the film and then expand outward. Another approach is looking from outside and then work in. Whatever approach you use, make sure you evaluate the following structures: cardiac shadows, lung fields, mediastinum, costophrenic angles, soft tissue, and bone. If there are any abnormalities noted, make sure you compare them with old films. Here are a few basic chest x-ray findings that you need to know.

The Cardiac Silhouette

On the **PA** or **AP** film:

Right heart border	⇨	**Right Atrium**
Left heart border	⇨	**Left Atrium** (superiorly) and **Left Ventricle** (inferiorly)

On the **lateral** film:

Part of the heart closest to the sternum	⇨	**Right Ventricle**
Part of the heart closest to the spine	⇨	**Left Atrium** (superiorly) and **Left Ventricle** (inferiorly and sitting on the diaphragm)

Silhouette Signs

Silhouette signs are present when the normal radiographic borders are lost. Changes in air/water densities from physiologic or disease processes cause these signs. The following are common positive silhouette signs that you will encounter.

Loss of	⇨	Represents
Right heart border	⇨	Right middle lobe abnormality
Left heart border	⇨	Lingula abnormality
Right hemidiaphragm	⇨	Right lower lobe abnormality
Left hemidiaphragm	⇨	Left lower lobe abnormality

Other signs

	⇨	
Blunting of the costophrenic angle	⇨	Pleural effusion
Air bronchograms	⇨	Fluid (pus, blood, edema) in the alveoli
Kerley B lines	⇨	Fluid in the interlobular septa

Appendix F: Common Abbreviations

Reading a chart can be very difficult if you do not know what the abbreviations or acronyms represent. The following are common, well accepted abbreviations and acronyms that you may encounter when you review a patient's chart.

	Seen in the History
AAA	abdominal aortic aneurysm
AMS	altered mental status
AMI	acute myocardial infarction
BPH	benign prostatic hypertrophy
Bx	biopsy
CABG	coronary artery bypass graft
CAD	coronary artery disease
c̄	with
c/o	complaining of
CVA	cerebral vascular accident, aka "stroke"
DJD	degenerative joint disease
DOE	dyspnea on exertion
ESRD	end stage renal disease
GERD	gastroesophageal reflux disease
HTN	hypertension
I&D	incision and drainage
IVDA	intravenous drug abuse
NKDA	no known drug allergies
PCN	penicillin
PCI	percutaneous coronary intervention
PND	paroxysmal nocturnal dyspnea
PTA	prior to admission
PTCA	percutaneous transluminal coronary angioplasty
s̄	without
s/p	status post - after ("post") an intervention)
x̄	except

Seen in Medications

ATC	around the clock
bid	twice daily
IM	intramuscular
IV	intravenous
PO	orally
PR	rectally
q	every
q4h	every 4 hours
qAC	before every meal
qAM	every morning
qD	every day
qHS	before bedtime every day
qid	four times daily
qOD	every other day
qPM	every evening
SC	subcutaneous
tid	three times daily

Seen in the Physical Exam

General

NAD   no apparent distress

HEENT

NC/AT   normocephalic/atraumatic
PERRLA pupil equally round and reactive to light and accommodation
EOMI   extra-ocular muscles intact
MMM   moist mucous membrane

Neck

JVD   jugular venous distention
LAD   lymphadenopathy

CV

RRR   regular rate and rhythm
m/g/r   murmurs/gallops/rubs

Lungs

CTAB   clear to auscultation bilaterally

Abdomen

NT/ND   nontender/nondistended
NABS   normoactive bowel sounds
HSM   hepatosplenomegaly

Extremities

C/C/E   clubbing/cyanosis/edema

Wounds

C/D/I   clean/dry/intact

Appendix G: Important Numbers

Here is a list of some important numbers that you want to keep handy. Have it in your PDA or in your pocket at all times.

Team Members

Resident Name: Pager:

Intern #1:   Pager:

Intern #2:   Pager:

Attending: Office No:

                                        Other No:

Co-Student: Pager:

Co-Student: Pager:

Other: Pager:

Services

Chemistry: Hematology:

Microbiology: Radiology:

Dictated Reports:

Gen Radiology (Xrays):

CT:

MRI:

Miscellaneous

EKG:

Transportation:.

Social Work:

Medicine Office #

Dean's Office #

Nursing Units

Telemetry Unit:

Appendix H: Patient Data Template

Here is a list of some of the things you want to keep track of regarding your patients. A template has been provided for you to use, or you can create your own template to suit your needs.

Patient Information

Identification
- Name
- Medical Record Number
- Contact and Contact Numbers
- Location
- Date of Admission

History
- Chief Complaint
- HPI
- PMH
- PSH
- FH
- SH
- Medications (outpatient and inpatient)
- Allergies
- ROS

Physical
- Vital Signs
- Physical Exam

Labs
- CBC
- Electrolytes
- Liver Function Tests
- Cardiac Enzymes
- Urine Studies
- Culture Results

Studies
- CXR
- EKG

Name: MR#:	Date: Room:	Allergies:
CC: HPI: ROS: ER:	Contact #s:	
	Diagnosis: Problem List:	
PMH:　　　　FH: SH: PSH	Meds Outpt:	Meds Inpt:
PE:	Misc.:	

APPENDIX H: PATIENT DATA TEMPLATE

Date	BP	P	T	R

Set	CK	Mb	Trop
1			
2			
3			

Studies:

Date			
WBC			
H/H			
Plts			
Na			
K			
Cl			
HCO3			
BUN			
Cr			
Glu			
Ca			
Mg			
Phos			
Tprot			
Alb			
Tbil			
Dbil			
ALP			
AST			
ALT			
PT/INR			

Cultures:

UA:

Clinician's Guide to Diagnosis

ISBN #1930598513

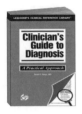

The work-up of a newly admitted patient is challenging for most students. Whereas students have learned about various diseases during the basic science years, patients, of course, do not present to the hospital saying they have one disease or another. Instead, patients present with symptoms and it is up to the student to determine which one of the diseases in the differential diagnosis is the cause of the symptom. During the patient evaluation, students are often unsure of what to ask in the history, what to look for in the physical exam, how to interpret abnormal lab test results, and how to put all this information together to come up with the patient's diagnosis.

These are precisely the questions for which the *Clinician's Guide to Diagnosis* provides the answers to. It is the only book that will lead you from symptom to diagnosis through a series of steps designed to mimic the logical thought processes of seasoned clinicians. For students, this is an ideal book to help bridge the gap between the classroom and actual patient care. It's truly a resource that can make a significant difference during your Internal Medicine clerkship. But don't take our word for it. See what others have had to say:

"I showed the book to one of my attendings. He said that it's one of the best books written for students and residents that he has ever seen. I'm not kidding you!"—Niraj Mehta, resident at Park Plaza Hospital

"This book serves as a worthy guide to a stepwise approach to common diagnoses. The information is presented in a simple to follow manner. It is intended to provide a practical approach to commonly encountered symptoms, a worthy objective that the book meets. Medical students and house officers are the intended audience. I would add primary care physicians. The author provides a unique step-by-step approach to the diagnosis of common problems. Tables and flowcharts are very well done. As a primary care physician, I am impressed with how easy it is to use this quick reference during a busy schedule."—Peter M. Daher, MD, Assistant Professor, Creighton University Medical Center (Doody Health Sciences Review)

"Samir Desai's text, *Clinician's Guide to Diagnosis: A Practical Approach,* provides a fresh approach to the ill patient because it is symptom-based not disease-based. The vast majority of texts assume the clinician already has arrived at a diagnosis and then provides information about that disease. However, if the diagnosis is unclear, the practitioner might have to read through many different disease entities to see which disease his/her patient's presentation most closely matches. This text takes a ground up approach, starting with the patient's symptoms and then working through the diagnosis. This book will be a helpful compendium not only for students and residents, but also for the senior clinician. I intend to consult it the next time I'm given an impossible CPC to solve."—Blasé A. Carabello, MD, Chief Medical Service, Veterans Affairs Medical Center, Houston, Texas

View a sample chapter at www.MD2B.net

Clinician's Guide to Internal Medicine ISBN # 159195021X

The Clinician's Guide to Internal Medicine provides quick access to essential information covering diagnosis, treatment, and management of commonly encountered problems in Internal Medicine. As a student, you'll find:

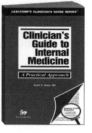

- Up-to-date information in an easy-to-read format

- Clinically relevant information that is easily accessible

- Practical approaches that are not readily available in standard textbooks

- Algorithms to help you establish the diagnosis and select the appropriate therapy

- Numerous tables and boxes that summarize diagnostic and therapeutic strategies

- Ideal reference for use at the point-of-care

Let the *Clinician's Guide to Internal Medicine: A Practical Approach* become your companion, providing you with the tools necessary to tackle even the most challenging problems in Internal Medicine.

View a sample chapter at www.MD2B.net

Clinician's Guide to Laboratory Medicine
2nd edition ISBN # 1930598742

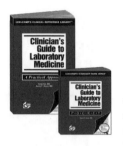

The *Clinician's Guide to Laboratory Medicine* is widely used by students and residents because it is the only book that provides practical approaches to lab test interpretation. Nowhere else will you find step-by-step approaches that will lead you from abnormal lab test to diagnosis. If you are having difficulty interpreting abnormal lab test results, determining what the next step is, or answering your attending physician's questions, this is the book that you need. But don't take our word for it. See what others have had to say:

"An excellent resource for medical students and residents... For example, the hyponatremia section is more useful than the one in the Wash manual... As they say on the wards, "Strong work!'" —Marc Levsky, during his 4th year of medical school at Northwestern University

"I shared the book with some of the residents that I am working with in Family Medicine. They love the book and are going to order it...They like the way the book is set up since it gives you what to look for when looking at lab results in a concise way...Your book will be a success!" —Damary Gonzalez, during his 3rd year of medical school at University of Illinois-Chicago

"Your text is wonderful... I have used it quite extensively on my medicine and surgical rotations during the last four months of my third year ... Many of my classmates and residents have even asked to borrow it."—Nicholas Mast, during his 3rd year of medical school at University of Nevada medical school

"My vote goes to the *Clinician's Guide to Laboratory Medicine: A Practical Approach.* by Desai. Pocket size, organized by chapters but in a question/answer format, with many algorithms to boot, reasonably priced. All the residents who ever saw my copy wrote down the name to buy one. I have Bakerman's and Wallach and used to have *The Right Test,* so I feel I have some ability to compare Desai's to other popular lab test books. Bakerman's and Wallach's have their place, but I would not even consider carrying either in my bag for a rotation."—Comment on the Student Doctor Network (www.studentdoctor.net) in response to a message inquiring about good lab test guides

"In our Medicine Clerkship, the *Clinician's Guide to Lab Medicine* has quickly become one of the two most popular paperback books that our students purchase for our clerkship. They also use it for other clerkships. Our students have praised the algorithms, tables, and ease of pursuit of clinical problems through better understanding of the utilization of tests appropriate to the problem at hand." —Gregory Magarian, MD, Director, 3rd Year Medicine Clerkship at Oregon Health Sciences University

View a sample chapter at www.MD2B.net

101 Biggest Mistakes 3rd Year Medical Students Make and How to Avoid Them

ISBN # 0-9725561-0-9

Compiled from discussions with hundreds of attending physicians, residents, and students, the *101 Biggest Mistakes 3rd Year Medical Students Make And How To Avoid Them* discusses the major mistakes that students make during this very important year. Avoiding these pitfalls is the key to third year success. This book will empower you, placing you in a position to have a successful experience, no matter what rotation or clerkship you are on. Once you are aware of the mistakes that students make, you can do everything in your power to avoid them, thereby becoming the savvy student that is poised for clerkship success. But don't take our word for it. See what others have had to say:

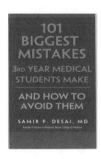

"Fear! That's the only way I can describe how I felt when I started my clinical clerkships. At our med school, we had a clinical orientation that was very basic. It really didn't help me get comfortable in the hospital setting. In my opinion, that's the key. Once you get comfortable in the hospital and know what your role/responsibilities are, then you have a chance to show the residents and attendings your best work. This book is unique in that it gives you a behind the scenes look at what attendings and residents are looking for in their students. By showing me the mistakes that students commonly make, I was able to avoid making the same ones. This helped me get great clinical evals and strong letters of recommendation, which are the keys to getting into the residency you want. I can't say enough about this book. I am convinced that it's one of the biggest reasons I honored so many of my rotations."—Review posted on www.bn.com.

"The third year of medical school is a difficult one. While the student is at last working in a clinical environment, each rotation brings a new series of experiences and emotions. Students have spent the last two years learning the basic science and are now faced with real life clinical experiences, which are exciting, frustrating, challenging and stressful. Each rotation is similar to beginning a new job, and it is not always apparent just what are the best ways to quickly and effectively adapt to the new fast paced demands, long hours and new responsibilities. Since the third year grades carry a heavy weight when a student is applying for a residency program it is very important to do as well as possible. Compiled from discussions with hundreds of attending physicians, residents, and students, this book shows you the 101 all-too-common mistakes students make. It also shows you how to avoid them so you don't fall into the same traps." — Excerpt from the MCW library website about the book, which was named the Medical College of Wisconsin Libraries Book of the Month (4/03)

View a sample chapter at www.MD2B.net

The Residency Match: 101 Biggest Mistakes and How to Avoid Them
ISBN # 0-9725561-1-7

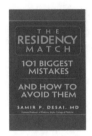

Are there any steps you can take to maximize your chances of matching with the residency program of your choice? One of the keys is to become familiar with the major mistakes that students make during the residency application process. These are mistakes that are well known to residency program directors but are not familiar to most applicants. In *The Residency Match: 101 Biggest Mistakes And How To Avoid Them*, we not only show you these mistakes but also help you avoid them, placing you in a position for match success. But don't take our word for it. See what others have had to say:

"The fourth year of medical school can be a stressful, demanding time. This books cuts down on the amount of necessary reading that you must do in order to match well. The book is a fast read that highlights the most important mistakes that others have made during the match process. It lets you in on tips on all subjects—from forming your CV to obtaining your letters of recommendation to developing your personal statement and preparing for interviews. I found the sections about the CV and personal statement very helpful and much easier to read than those same sections in a larger book about the match. The section on letters of recommendation was important because it directed me on the proper way to ask for and to attain the best letters of recommendation. The interview section contains good reminders of things that seem common sense but which you don't necessarily think about. It also has several tips about subjects I had not thought about (for example, you should have a case ready to present your interviewer), as well as questions you will be asked in interviews and questions you should ask the interviewer. Overall, this is an easy to read book that I would definitely recommend because it contains all the essentials to matching in your ideal residency spot."—Review posted by Jonathan Welch on www.amazon.com

View a sample chapter at www.MD2B.net